A Guide to Health and Happiness

25 Short Tales to Shape Up and Shed Pounds

Chapters:

Preface

1. **The Journey Begins: A Commitment to Change**

2. **Fitness Fundamentals: Getting Started**

3. **Workout Wonders: Transforming Your Body**

4. **Healthy Habits: Making Better Choices**

5. **Navigating Nutrition: Understanding Food**

6. **Diving into Diets: Finding What Works**

7. **Keto Kickstart: Embracing Ketogenic Eating**

8. **The Power of Caloric Deficit: Eating for Weight Loss**

9. **Mindful Eating: Being Present at the Table**

10. **Gender Differences in Weight Loss: Bridging the Gap**

11. **Hormones and Weight: Balancing the Equation**

12. **Muscles in Motion: Building Strength**

The End is Also A New Beggining

Preface:

Welcome to the transformative journey that lies within the pages of this book. As you embark on this exploration of health, wellness, and self-discovery, I invite you to open your mind and heart to the endless possibilities that await you.

The intention behind this book is simple yet profound: to empower you to become the happiest, healthiest version of yourself. In a world filled with conflicting information and quick-fix solutions, my aim is to provide you with a comprehensive guide that incorporates various diets, physical and mental wellness practices, fitness routines, and nutritional principles to support your journey towards holistic well-being.

Why such a broad scope, you may ask? Because true wellness encompasses so much more than just the number on a scale or the size of your waistline. It's about nurturing your body, mind, and spirit in harmony, creating a life filled with vitality, purpose, and joy.

Throughout these pages, you'll find a wealth of practical advice, evidence-based strategies, and inspirational stories to guide you on your path. Whether you're seeking to shed excess weight, boost your energy levels, improve your fitness, or simply enhance your overall quality of life, you'll find tools and resources here to support your goals.

But more than just a collection of tips and techniques, this book is a testament to the transformative power that lies within each and every one of us. It's a reminder that you have the ability to shape your destiny, to rewrite your story, and to become the architect of your own happiness.

As you journey through these pages, I encourage you to approach this process with an open mind and a spirit of curiosity. Embrace experimentation, celebrate progress, and be gentle with yourself along the way. Remember that change takes time, and that every step forward—no matter how small—is a victory worth celebrating.

Above all, know that you are not alone on this journey. I am here to support and guide you every step of the way, and I believe wholeheartedly in your ability to create the vibrant, fulfilling life that you deserve.

So let us embark on this adventure together, with hearts open and spirits soaring, as we discover the transformative power of health, wellness, and self-discovery. Here's to your journey towards becoming the happiest, healthiest version of yourself.

Chapter 1: The Journey Begins: A Commitment to Change

In a bustling town nestled between rolling hills and serene forests, there lived a woman named Emma. Emma was like many others in her community – kind-hearted, hardworking, and deeply yearning for a happier, healthier life. However, despite her genuine desire for change, Emma found herself overwhelmed by self-doubt, uncertainty, and a lack of knowledge about where to begin her journey.

One day, as she sat alone in her cozy apartment, feeling lost and unsure of her next steps, Emma stumbled upon a story titled "The Journey Begins: A Commitment to Change." Intrigued by the promise of guidance and support, Emma eagerly flipped through its pages, unsure of what to expect.

What she found inside was nothing short of a revelation. The story was filled with real-life examoles of individuals who had overcome their own struggles and transformed their lives for the better. From weight loss success stories to tales of personal growth and self-discovery, each story served as a beacon of hope and

inspiration for Emma, showing her that change was possible –
even in the face of doubt and uncertainty.

But the book offered more than just stories; it also provided
practical advice, tips, and resources for embarking on a journey of
personal transformation. From expert advice on nutrition and
exercise to strategies for building confidence and resilience, the
book gave Emma the tools she needed to take control of her health
and well-being.

As she delved deeper into the pages of the book, Emma felt a sense
of empowerment and clarity wash over her. She realized that she
didn't have to navigate her journey alone – that there were people
out there who understood her struggles and were willing to offer
guidance and support every step of the way.

Armed with newfound knowledge and confidence, Emma made a
commitment to herself to embrace change and embark on a journey
of self-discovery and transformation. She set small, achievable
goals for herself – whether it was incorporating more fruits and
vegetables into her diet, going for a daily walk, or practicing
mindfulness meditation – and celebrated each small victory along
the way.

And as she continued on her journey, Emma began to experience profound shifts in both her mental and physical well-being. She found joy in nourishing her body with wholesome foods, strength in challenging herself with new workouts, and peace in the quiet moments of reflection and self-care.

But perhaps the greatest transformation of all was the newfound sense of confidence and self-assurance that Emma gained through her journey. She learned to trust herself, to listen to her body's needs, and to believe in her ability to create the life she truly desired.

As Emma closed the book and looked out at the world around her, she knew that her journey was just beginning. But with the guidance and support she had found within its pages, she felt confident that she had everything she needed to navigate the challenges and obstacles that lay ahead.

And as she took the first steps on her journey, Emma couldn't help but feel a sense of gratitude for the book that had helped her find her way. It had been more than just a collection of words on a page – it had been a lifeline, a source of inspiration, and a guiding light on her path to a happier, healthier life.

Short Story: The Decision

Amelia sat on her couch, scrolling through old photos on her phone. She came across a picture from a few years ago—a time when she felt healthier, more energetic, and confident in her own skin. Looking at herself now, she realized how much she had let herself go. Stress, a busy schedule, and a lack of self-care had taken their toll. But in that moment, something clicked. She made a decision—a commitment to change.

Section 1: Recognizing the Need for Change

Making the decision to embark on a weight loss journey often begins with a moment of realization. Whether it's seeing an old photograph, struggling to keep up with daily activities, or experiencing health concerns, recognizing the need for change is the first step towards a healthier lifestyle.

Practical Tips:

1. Reflect on your current habits and how they impact your overall well-being.

2. Identify specific areas where you want to see improvement, whether it's weight loss, increased energy, or better health.

3. Set realistic goals that are achievable and sustainable in the long term.

Section 2: Setting Intentions

Once you've acknowledged the need for change, it's essential to set clear intentions for your journey. Define what success looks like for you and establish your reasons for wanting to lose weight. Whether it's improving your health, boosting your confidence, or increasing your quality of life, your intentions will guide your actions moving forward.

Practical Tips:

1. Write down your reasons for wanting to lose weight and revisit them regularly for motivation.

2. Set specific, measurable, achievable, relevant, and time-bound (SMART) goals to keep you focused and on track.

3. Visualize yourself achieving your goals and imagine how your life will improve as a result.

Section 3: Building a Support System

Embarking on a weight loss journey can be challenging, but you don't have to do it alone. Surround yourself with supportive friends, family members, or peers who will encourage and motivate you along the way. Building a strong support system can provide accountability, guidance, and emotional support during both the ups and downs of your journey.

Practical Tips:

1. Share your goals with trusted individuals who will cheer you on and hold you accountable.
2. Seek out online communities, support groups, or fitness classes where you can connect with others who are on a similar path.
3. Don't be afraid to ask for help when you need it, whether it's assistance with meal planning, workout advice, or emotional support.

Section 4: Embracing a Growth Mindset

As you embark on your weight loss journey, it's important to adopt a growth mindset—a belief that your abilities and intelligence can be developed through dedication and hard work. Instead of viewing setbacks as failures, see them as opportunities for growth and learning. Approach challenges with resilience, perseverance, and a willingness to adapt your strategies as needed.

Practical Tips:

1. Focus on progress rather than perfection, celebrating small victories along the way.
2. Embrace challenges as opportunities to learn and grow stronger.
3. Practice self-compassion and kindness towards yourself, especially during difficult moments.

Section 5: Taking the First Steps

With your intentions set and support system in place, it's time to take the first steps towards your weight loss goals. Start by making small, manageable changes to your daily habits, such as incorporating more fruits and vegetables into your meals, finding enjoyable forms of physical activity, and prioritizing self-care practices that nourish your body and mind.

Practical Tips:

1. Start with achievable goals, such as walking for 30 minutes a day or replacing sugary drinks with water.
2. Experiment with different forms of exercise to find activities that you enjoy and look forward to.
3. Be patient and persistent, remembering that lasting change takes time and effort.

By recognizing the need for change, setting clear intentions, building a support system, embracing a growth mindset, and taking the first steps towards your goals, you're laying the foundation for a successful weight loss journey. Remember, every step you take brings you closer to the healthier, happier life you deserve.

Chapter 2: Fitness Fundamentals: Getting Started

Introducing Jason, a 34-year-old man who found himself at a crossroads in life. As he looked in the mirror one morning, he couldn't help but feel dissatisfied with the reflection staring back at him. Years of neglecting his health and fitness had taken their toll, leaving him feeling sluggish, overweight, and out of shape.

Despite his desire to make a change, Jason felt overwhelmed by the prospect of starting a fitness journey. He had no idea where to begin or how to navigate the world of exercise and nutrition. Doubts and insecurities crept into his mind, whispering that he was too old, too out of shape, too busy to embark on such a daunting endeavor.

But deep down, Jason knew that he couldn't continue living life on autopilot. He longed to reclaim his vitality, to feel strong and confident in his own skin once again. And so, with a mixture of trepidation and determination, he made the decision to take the first step towards a healthier, happier life.

Armed with a newfound sense of purpose, Jason began his journey by educating himself on the fundamentals of fitness. He devoured articles, watched videos, and sought advice from friends and family who had experience in the world of exercise. Slowly but surely, he started to piece together the puzzle of what it meant to live a healthy, active lifestyle.

One of the first lessons Jason learned was the importance of setting realistic goals. Instead of fixating on grandiose visions of six-pack abs and marathon finishes, he focused on achievable objectives that would keep him motivated and on track. Whether it was losing a few pounds, running a mile without stopping, or simply feeling more energized throughout the day, Jason knew that every small victory brought him one step closer to his ultimate goal.

With his goals in mind, Jason turned his attention to creating a workout routine that suited his lifestyle and fitness level. He started with simple, beginner-friendly exercises that required minimal equipment, such as bodyweight squats, push-ups, and lunges. Gradually, he began to incorporate more challenging workouts, experimenting with different forms of exercise to keep things interesting and engaging.

As Jason immersed himself in his newfound fitness routine, he was amazed by the changes he began to see and feel in his body. His energy levels soared, his mood lifted, and he discovered a newfound sense of strength and confidence that he hadn't felt in years. Gone were the days of sluggishness and self-doubt; in their place stood a man who was determined, resilient, and ready to take on the world.

But perhaps the greatest transformation of all was the shift that took place within Jason's mind and spirit. As he pushed himself to new heights and conquered obstacles he once thought insurmountable, he gained a newfound sense of self-belief and resilience. He learned to embrace the journey, to celebrate progress over perfection, and to trust in his own ability to overcome any challenge that came his way.

Today, Jason stands as a shining example of the transformative power of fitness fundamentals. He has not only transformed his body but also his mind and spirit, emerging stronger, happier, and more confident than ever before. And though his journey is far from over, he knows that as long as he continues to show up, put in the work, and believe in himself, the possibilities for growth and transformation are endless.

Short Story: The First Workout

Jake stood in front of the gym entrance, feeling a mix of excitement and nervousness. He had made a commitment to prioritize his health and fitness, and today was the day he would take the first step towards that goal. With determination in his heart, he walked through the doors and into a world of possibilities.

Section 1: Understanding the Importance of Fitness

Fitness is not just about looking good; it's about feeling good, both physically and mentally. Regular physical activity has numerous benefits, including improved cardiovascular health, increased strength and endurance, enhanced mood, and reduced risk of chronic diseases. By prioritizing fitness, you're investing in your overall well-being and longevity.

Practical Tips:

1. Educate yourself about the benefits of exercise and how it can positively impact your life.
2. Set clear fitness goals that align with your overall health objectives.
3. Start slowly and gradually increase the intensity and duration of your workouts as your fitness level improves.

Section 2: Finding Your Why

Before diving into a fitness routine, it's essential to understand your motivation behind wanting to get fit. Whether it's improving your physical health, boosting your confidence, relieving stress, or setting a positive example for your loved ones, clarifying your reasons for wanting to exercise will help you stay focused and committed when faced with challenges.

Practical Tips:

1. Take some time to reflect on your personal reasons for wanting to get fit.
2. Write down your fitness goals and the benefits you hope to achieve from regular exercise.
3. Remind yourself of your why whenever you feel unmotivated or discouraged.

Section 3: Starting Small

Embarking on a fitness journey can feel overwhelming, especially if you're new to exercise or haven't been active in a while. Instead of trying to do too much too soon, focus on starting small and gradually building momentum over time. Consistency is key, and small, sustainable changes can lead to significant results in the long run.

Practical Tips:

1. Begin with activities that you enjoy and feel comfortable doing, such as walking, swimming, or cycling.
2. Start with short workout sessions and gradually increase the duration and intensity as your fitness level improves.
3. Break your fitness goals into smaller, manageable milestones to track your progress and celebrate your achievements along the way.

Section 4: Setting Up Your Fitness Plan

A well-rounded fitness plan includes a combination of cardiovascular exercise, strength training, flexibility work, and restorative practices. Designing a plan that incorporates a variety of activities will help you develop a balanced physique, prevent boredom, and reduce the risk of overuse injuries. Additionally, consider factors such as your fitness level, preferences, schedule, and access to equipment when creating your plan.

Practical Tips:

1. Consult with a fitness professional to help you design a personalized workout plan based on your goals and abilities.
2. Incorporate a mix of aerobic, strength, and flexibility exercises into your routine for comprehensive fitness benefits.
3. Schedule your workouts like appointments, prioritizing consistency and making exercise a non-negotiable part of your day.

Section 5: Listen to Your Body

One of the most important aspects of fitness is learning to listen to your body's cues and signals. Pay attention to how you feel during and after exercise, and adjust your intensity, duration, and type of activity accordingly. Remember that rest and recovery are just as important as physical activity, allowing your body to heal, repair, and adapt to the demands of exercise.

Practical Tips:

1. Start each workout with a proper warm-up to prepare your body for exercise and reduce the risk of injury.
2. Pay attention to any pain or discomfort during exercise and modify or stop activities that cause pain.
3. Incorporate rest days into your fitness routine to allow your body to recover and prevent burnout or overtraining.

By understanding the importance of fitness, clarifying your motivation, starting small, designing a personalized fitness plan, and listening to your body, you're laying the groundwork for a successful journey towards improved health and vitality. Remember, every step you take towards a fitter, stronger you is a step in the right direction.

Chapter 3: Workout Wonders: Transforming Your Body

In the realm of fitness and health, this mantra has become a guiding principle for many individuals embarking on their journey towards weight loss. It encapsulates the idea that consistency and effort are key components of success, emphasizing the importance of showing up and putting in the work, regardless of the circumstances.

In this chapter, we delve into the significance of this mindset and explore how adopting it can propel you closer to your fitness goals. We'll uncover the psychological and physiological benefits of regular exercise, debunk common myths surrounding workouts, and provide practical strategies for overcoming barriers to consistency.

Emily's Journey From Inertia to Action

Once upon a time, there lived a woman named Emily who found herself stuck in a rut of unhealthy habits and sedentary lifestyle. At 30 years old, she worked a demanding office job that kept her glued to her desk for long hours, leaving little time for physical activity. Her diet consisted mainly of convenience foods and takeout meals, and stress from work often led her to indulge in mindless snacking and emotional eating.

Despite her longing for change, Emily struggled to find the motivation and energy to break free from her unhealthy habits. She felt trapped in a cycle of lethargy and self-doubt, unsure of where to begin her journey towards a healthier, more active life.

One day, while browsing through social media, Emily stumbled upon a post that caught her eye: "The only bad workout is the one that didn't happen." Intrigued by the message, she delved deeper into the world of fitness and discovered a wealth of inspiring stories and practical tips for incorporating exercise into her daily routine.

Determined to make a change, Emily decided to start small. She began by setting aside just 30 minutes each day for physical activity, whether it was a brisk walk around the neighborhood, a yoga session in her living room, or a quick workout at the gym. Despite her initial doubts and insecurities, Emily pushed through the discomfort and embraced the challenge of moving her body every day.

As the days turned into weeks, Emily started to notice subtle changes taking place within herself. She felt more energized and alert throughout the day, and her mood lifted as she experienced the endorphin rush that came with regular exercise. Gradually, she began to shed the excess weight that had been weighing her down for so long, and her confidence soared as she saw her body becoming stronger and more toned.

But perhaps the most profound transformation took place within Emily's mind and spirit. With each workout she completed, she gained a newfound sense of accomplishment and self-worth. She learned to push through her limits and embrace the discomfort of physical exertion, knowing that each drop of sweat was a testament to her commitment to change.

As Emily's journey progressed, she discovered a newfound passion for fitness and a deep appreciation for her body's capabilities. She found joy in the simple act of movement, whether it was dancing to her favorite music, hiking through nature, or trying out new workout classes with friends. Exercise became not just a chore, but a source of joy, empowerment, and self-discovery.

Today, Emily stands tall as a shining example of the transformative power of regular physical activity. She has overcome the barriers of laziness and self-doubt to become the healthiest, happiest version of herself. And though her journey is far from over, she knows that as long as she keeps showing up and putting in the work, the possibilities for growth and transformation are endless.

For Emily, the mantra "The only bad workout is the one that didn't happen" serves as a reminder of her journey from inertia to action, from doubt to determination. It is a testament to the power of consistency, perseverance, and belief in oneself. And as she continues on her path towards greater health and vitality, Emily knows that with each workout she completes, she is one step closer to becoming the best version of herself.

The Power of Consistency:

Consistency is the cornerstone of any successful fitness regimen. Whether you're aiming to shed excess pounds, build strength, or improve overall health, committing to regular exercise is essential for long-term progress. Consistent workouts not only help you develop physical strength and endurance but also cultivate discipline, resilience, and a sense of accomplishment.

The Myth of Perfection:

One of the biggest misconceptions about exercise is the notion that every workout must be intense and flawless to yield results. In reality, progress is not linear, and setbacks are inevitable. Embracing the idea that imperfect workouts still contribute to your overall progress can alleviate pressure and foster a healthier relationship with fitness.

Overcoming Barriers to Consistency:

Maintaining a consistent workout routine can be challenging, especially in the face of busy schedules, fatigue, and lack of motivation. However, by identifying and addressing common barriers to consistency, such as time constraints, boredom, and self-doubt, you can develop strategies to stay on track and overcome obstacles along the way.

Practical Strategies for Success:

To ensure that every workout counts, it's essential to prioritize quality over quantity and focus on sustainable habits that align with your goals and lifestyle. Whether it's finding activities you enjoy, scheduling workouts in advance, or enlisting the support of a workout buddy, there are numerous strategies you can employ to stay consistent and motivated on your fitness journey.

Celebrating Progress, Not Perfection:

Finally, it's crucial to celebrate your efforts and progress, no matter how small. By shifting your focus from perfection to progress, you can cultivate a positive mindset and stay motivated to continue pushing towards your goals. Remember, every workout—even the ones that don't go as planned—is a step in the right direction.

In the end, adopting the mindset that "the only bad workout is the one that didn't happen" empowers you to prioritize consistency, embrace imperfection, and stay committed to your fitness journey. By showing up and putting in the work, day in and day out, you'll not only transform your body but also cultivate resilience, discipline, and a deep sense of personal empowerment. So lace up your sneakers, hit the gym, and remember: every workout brings you one step closer to becoming the best version of yourself.

Here are some evidence-based examples of how various levels of exercise benefit the body and contribute to weight loss compared to a sedentary lifestyle:

1. **Cardiovascular Health:** Regular aerobic exercise, such as brisk walking, running, swimming, or cycling, has been shown to improve cardiovascular health by strengthening the heart and improving circulation. Studies have found that individuals who engage in moderate to vigorous aerobic activity have a lower risk of developing heart disease, stroke, and high blood pressure compared to those who are sedentary.

2. **Weight Management:** Engaging in regular physical activity helps to burn calories, which is essential for weight management. Both aerobic exercise and strength training can contribute to weight loss by increasing metabolic rate and building lean muscle mass. Research has shown that individuals who exercise regularly are more likely to achieve and maintain a healthy weight compared to those who are inactive.

3. **Metabolic Health:** Exercise plays a crucial role in improving metabolic health by increasing insulin sensitivity and reducing the risk of type 2 diabetes. Even moderate levels of physical activity, such as walking or gardening, have been shown to lower blood sugar levels and improve insulin response. Incorporating regular exercise into your

routine can help regulate blood sugar levels and reduce the risk of metabolic disorders.

4. **Muscle Strength and Function:** Strength training exercises, such as weightlifting or resistance training, help to build and maintain muscle mass, which is important for overall health and function. As we age, muscle mass naturally declines, leading to decreased strength, mobility, and independence. Regular strength training can counteract age-related muscle loss and improve muscle strength, endurance, and function.

5. **Bone Health:** Weight-bearing exercises, such as walking, jogging, or dancing, help to strengthen bones and reduce the risk of osteoporosis. Studies have shown that regular exercise stimulates bone formation and increases bone density, reducing the risk of fractures and bone-related injuries. Incorporating weight-bearing exercises into your routine can help maintain bone health and prevent age-related bone loss.

6. **Mental Health:** Exercise has been shown to have numerous mental health benefits, including reducing symptoms of depression, anxiety, and stress. Physical activity stimulates the release of endorphins,

neurotransmitters that promote feelings of happiness and well-being. Additionally, regular exercise improves sleep quality, cognitive function, and overall mood, leading to better mental health outcomes.

7. **Longevity:** Numerous studies have found a strong association between regular physical activity and increased longevity. Engaging in regular exercise has been shown to reduce the risk of premature death from all causes, including heart disease, cancer, and other chronic conditions. Adopting an active lifestyle can significantly improve overall health and longevity, allowing you to live a longer, healthier life.

In summary, regular exercise offers a myriad of benefits for both physical and mental health, including improved cardiovascular health, weight management, metabolic health, muscle strength, bone health, mental well-being, and longevity. Compared to a sedentary lifestyle, incorporating various levels of physical activity into your routine can significantly improve overall health outcomes and contribute to successful weight loss and weight management.

Getting Off the Couch it Could Save Your Life

A sedentary lifestyle, characterized by a lack of regular physical activity, poses numerous risks to both physical and mental health. One of the primary concerns associated with not exercising regularly is an increased risk of developing chronic health conditions. Without adequate physical activity, individuals are more susceptible to obesity, cardiovascular disease, type 2 diabetes, hypertension, and metabolic syndrome. Prolonged periods of inactivity can lead to weight gain, particularly visceral fat accumulation around organs, which further elevates the risk of chronic diseases.

Moreover, a lack of regular exercise can have detrimental effects on cardiovascular health. Physical inactivity contributes to poor circulation, reduced heart function, and an increased risk of heart disease and stroke. Without the stimulus of regular exercise, the heart muscles weaken over time, compromising its ability to pump blood efficiently and increasing the likelihood of cardiovascular events.

Muscle weakness and loss of muscle mass are also common consequences of a sedentary lifestyle. Without regular physical activity, muscles become deconditioned and lose strength and tone, leading to decreased mobility, flexibility, and balance. This can increase the risk of falls, fractures, and mobility-related issues, particularly in older adults.

In addition to physical health risks, a sedentary lifestyle is associated with adverse mental health outcomes. Lack of exercise has been linked to an increased risk of depression, anxiety, and stress. Physical activity stimulates the release of endorphins, neurotransmitters that promote feelings of happiness and well-being. Without regular exercise, individuals may experience mood disturbances, reduced cognitive function, and decreased overall quality of life.

Furthermore, a sedentary lifestyle contributes to a higher risk of premature mortality. Studies have consistently shown that individuals who engage in regular physical activity have a lower risk of death from all causes compared to those who are inactive. Physical inactivity is considered a significant risk factor for premature death, highlighting the importance of regular exercise for longevity and overall health.

The potential risks of not exercising regularly are numerous and far-reaching, encompassing both physical and mental health. From an increased risk of chronic diseases and cardiovascular events to muscle weakness, depression, and premature mortality, the consequences of a sedentary lifestyle are profound. Prioritizing regular physical activity is essential for maintaining optimal health and well-being throughout life.

Even small amounts of physical activity each week can offer significant health benefits compared to individuals who never exercise. Research has consistently shown that incorporating even brief periods of movement into one's routine can have a profound impact on overall health and well-being. For example, engaging in as little as 150 minutes of moderate-intensity aerobic activity per week—equivalent to just 30 minutes a day, five days a week—has been associated with reduced risk of chronic diseases such as heart disease, type 2 diabetes, and certain types of cancer. These benefits extend beyond physical health, as regular exercise has also been linked to improved mental health outcomes, including reduced symptoms of depression, anxiety, and stress.

Additionally, small amounts of physical activity can contribute to better sleep quality, increased energy levels, and enhanced cognitive function. By simply incorporating short bouts of movement into daily life, individuals can experience a multitude of benefits that significantly improve overall health and quality of life, even compared to those who remain sedentary.

Chapter 4: Healthy Habits: Making Better Choices

Meet Sarah, a 35-year-old marketing executive who struggled with a sedentary lifestyle, poor dietary habits, and stress-related eating. For years, Sarah found herself caught in a cycle of long work hours, fast food meals, and emotional eating to cope with the demands of her job. As a result, she had gained excess weight, felt constantly fatigued, and experienced frequent mood swings and anxiety.

However, Sarah reached a turning point when she realized that her unhealthy habits were taking a toll on her physical and mental well-being. Determined to make a change, she embarked on a journey to transform her lifestyle and prioritize her health.

Sarah began by incorporating regular exercise into her daily routine. Despite her busy schedule, she committed to taking short walks during her lunch break and attending yoga classes in the evenings. Gradually, she started to notice improvements in her energy levels, mood, and overall fitness. With time, Sarah's workouts became a source of stress relief and empowerment, rather than a chore.

In addition to exercise, Sarah revamped her diet, opting for nutritious, whole foods instead of processed snacks and fast food. She experimented with meal prepping on weekends, preparing healthy meals and snacks to enjoy throughout the week. By fueling her body with nutrient-dense foods, Sarah found that she had more energy, fewer cravings, and greater satisfaction from her meals.

As Sarah's physical health improved, so did her mental well-being. She discovered healthy ways to manage stress, such as practicing mindfulness meditation and prioritizing self-care activities like reading and spending time outdoors. With these tools, Sarah learned to cope with stress in a constructive manner, rather than turning to food for comfort.

Over time, Sarah's dedication to her health and well-being paid off in more ways than she could have imagined. Not only did she lose excess weight and achieve a healthier body composition, but she also experienced a profound transformation in her confidence, self-esteem, and overall outlook on life. She found joy in physical activity, nourished her body with wholesome foods, and cultivated a sense of balance and fulfillment that she had never known before.

Today, Sarah continues to prioritize her health and well-being, recognizing that self-care is not a luxury but a necessity for living a vibrant, fulfilling life. Through her journey, she serves as an inspiration to others, demonstrating that with commitment, perseverance, and self-love, anyone can overcome unhealthy habits and create a life filled with vitality, joy, and well-being.

Sarah's transformation began with a deep commitment to change and a willingness to confront her unhealthy habits head-on. She recognized that her sedentary lifestyle, poor dietary choices, and stress-related eating were not only affecting her physical health but also taking a toll on her mental and emotional well-being. Determined to make a positive change, Sarah took deliberate steps to overhaul her lifestyle and prioritize her health.

First and foremost, Sarah set clear and achievable goals for herself. She started small, incorporating simple changes into her daily routine, such as taking short walks during her lunch break and opting for healthier meal options. By setting realistic goals and focusing on gradual progress, Sarah was able to build momentum and maintain consistency in her efforts.

Additionally, Sarah sought out support and accountability from friends, family, and online communities. She shared her goals with loved ones, who offered encouragement, guidance, and practical tips for staying on track. Sarah also connected with like-minded individuals through online forums and social media groups, where she found inspiration, motivation, and a sense of camaraderie on her journey towards better health.

Furthermore, Sarah took a proactive approach to addressing the underlying causes of her unhealthy habits. She recognized that stress played a significant role in her eating patterns and sought out healthier ways to manage her emotions. Through mindfulness meditation, deep breathing exercises, and other stress-reduction techniques, Sarah learned to cope with stress in a constructive manner, rather than turning to food for comfort.

As Sarah began to see progress in her physical health and well-being, she experienced a shift in her mindset and perspective. She started to view exercise and healthy eating not as obligations but as opportunities to nurture and care for her body. With each healthy choice she made, Sarah felt a renewed sense of empowerment, confidence, and self-esteem.

Over time, Sarah's commitment to her health and well-being paid off in profound ways. She shed excess weight, gained strength and vitality, and achieved a greater sense of balance and fulfillment in her life. Through her journey, Sarah learned that change is possible, no matter how daunting the obstacles may seem, and that by taking small, consistent steps towards better health, anyone can create a life filled with vitality, joy, and well-being.

Here's a list of example bad habits and good habits to replace them with, along with their benefits:

Bad Habit: Sedentary Lifestyle

- Sitting for long periods without movement
- Lack of regular physical activity

Good Habit: Regular Exercise

- Engaging in aerobic exercise, strength training, or flexibility exercises

- Benefits: Improved cardiovascular health, increased muscle strength and endurance, better mood and mental health, weight management, reduced risk of chronic diseases

Bad Habit: Poor Dietary Choices

- Consuming high amounts of processed foods, sugary snacks, and fast food
- Skipping meals or eating irregularly

Good Habit: Balanced Diet

- Eating a variety of fruits, vegetables, lean proteins, whole grains, and healthy fats
- Incorporating regular meals and snacks to maintain energy levels
- Benefits: Provides essential nutrients for optimal health, supports weight management, reduces the risk of chronic diseases, improves energy levels and overall well-being

Bad Habit: Smoking

- Tobacco use, including cigarettes, cigars, or e-cigarettes
- Inhalation of harmful chemicals and toxins

Good Habit: Smoking Cessation

- Quitting smoking through behavioral interventions, nicotine replacement therapy, or prescription medications
- Seeking support from healthcare professionals, counselors, or support groups
- Benefits: Reduces the risk of cancer, heart disease, respiratory problems, and other tobacco-related diseases, improves lung function, increases life expectancy

Bad Habit: Excessive Alcohol Consumption

- Drinking alcohol in excess of recommended guidelines
- Binge drinking or frequent heavy drinking

Good Habit: Moderate Drinking

- Consuming alcohol in moderation, if at all
- Following recommended guidelines for moderate alcohol consumption (up to one drink per day for women and up to two drinks per day for men)

- Benefits: Reduces the risk of alcohol-related health problems, such as liver disease, heart disease, and certain cancers, promotes overall health and well-being

Bad Habit: Stress Eating

- Using food as a coping mechanism for stress, anxiety, or boredom
- Mindless eating or emotional eating in response to negative emotions

Good Habit: Stress Management

- Practicing stress-reduction techniques, such as mindfulness meditation, deep breathing exercises, or progressive muscle relaxation
- Finding healthy ways to cope with stress, such as exercise, hobbies, socializing, or creative outlets
- Benefits: Reduces stress levels, promotes relaxation and calmness, improves mood and mental well-being, prevents overeating and unhealthy eating habits

In conclusion, the benefits of changing bad habits extend far beyond physical health; they encompass every aspect of our lives, contributing to greater happiness, fulfillment, and overall well-being. By taking proactive steps to replace unhealthy behaviors with positive habits, individuals can transform their lives and unlock their full potential.

Embracing regular exercise not only strengthens our bodies and improves physical fitness but also boosts mood, enhances mental clarity, and instills a sense of empowerment. Making healthier dietary choices nourishes our bodies from the inside out, providing essential nutrients for optimal health and vitality. Quitting smoking and moderating alcohol consumption reduce the risk of serious diseases and improve longevity, while stress management techniques promote inner peace, resilience, and emotional balance.

As we cultivate healthy habits, we begin to experience a profound shift in our mindset and perspective. We gain a newfound sense of control over our lives, recognizing that we have the power to shape our destiny through the choices we make each day. With each positive change we implement, we move closer to our goals, whether they be achieving a healthy weight, overcoming addiction, or simply living a more vibrant and fulfilling life.

Ultimately, the journey towards changing bad habits is not always easy, but the rewards are immeasurable. By committing to our well-being and prioritizing self-care, we lay the foundation for a happier, healthier, and more fulfilling life. Through perseverance, determination, and a belief in our own potential, we can break free from the limitations of our past and step into a brighter future— one filled with vitality, joy, and boundless possibilities.

Chapter 5: Navigating Nutrition: Understanding Food

In a quaint suburban neighborhood, there lived a woman named Julia. Julia was a busy mother of two young children, juggling a full-time job, household responsibilities, and the demands of family life. Like many others in her community, Julia often found herself relying on convenience foods and takeout meals to feed her family, sacrificing nutrition for the sake of convenience.

Despite her best intentions, Julia couldn't shake the feeling that her family's diet was lacking in the nutrients needed to support their health and well-being. She noticed that her energy levels were inconsistent, her mood often fluctuated, and her children seemed to be constantly battling colds and infections.

Determined to make a change for the better, Julia embarked on a journey to educate herself about nutrition and make healthier choices for her family. She devoured books, articles, and online resources, soaking up information about the importance of whole foods, balanced meals, and mindful eating practices.

Armed with knowledge and determination, Julia set out to overhaul her family's diet, one meal at a time. She began by making simple swaps, such as replacing processed snacks with fresh fruits and vegetables, and trading sugary drinks for water or herbal tea. She experimented with new recipes and cooking methods, discovering the joy of preparing wholesome meals from scratch.

As Julia implemented these changes, she began to notice a remarkable transformation in her family's health and well-being. Her children's immune systems seemed stronger, and they were sick less often. Julia herself experienced more stable energy levels throughout the day, and her mood improved significantly.

But perhaps the most profound change of all was the impact on Julia's mental and emotional well-being. As she nourished her body with nutrient-rich foods, she found herself feeling more grounded, centered, and at peace with herself and the world around her. She discovered that food wasn't just fuel for the body – it was medicine for the mind and soul as well.

Inspired by Julia's journey, her neighbor Tom decided to take a closer look at his own diet and lifestyle choices. Tom was a middle-aged man who had spent years indulging in fast food, processed snacks, and sugary drinks. His sedentary lifestyle had led to weight gain, high cholesterol, and low energy levels, leaving him feeling lethargic and uninspired.

Determined to reclaim his health and vitality, Tom made the decision to overhaul his diet and incorporate regular exercise into his routine. He started by cutting out processed foods and sugary drinks, replacing them with whole, nutrient-rich foods such as fruits, vegetables, lean proteins, and whole grains.

Tom also began to prioritize physical activity, incorporating daily walks, bike rides, and strength training sessions into his schedule. As he shed excess weight and built strength and endurance, he noticed a significant improvement in his energy levels, mood, and overall sense of well-being.

Encouraged by his progress, Tom's wife Kim decided to join him on his journey to better health. Together, they supported and motivated each other, sharing healthy meals, trying out new recipes, and exploring different forms of exercise.

As Tom and Kim embraced their new lifestyle, they discovered a newfound sense of vitality and joy that they had never experienced before. They felt more connected to each other, more present in their daily lives, and more optimistic about the future.

And as they looked back on their journey, Tom and Kim realized that the key to their success had been a simple yet powerful realization: that food has the power to heal, nourish, and transform both body and soul. By making conscious choices about what they put into their bodies, they had unlocked a new level of health, happiness, and vitality – and they couldn't wait to see where their journey would take them next.

High salt and sugar diets can have significant negative impacts on our bodies, contributing to various health issues and hindering weight loss efforts. Here are some examples of how excessive salt and sugar intake can affect our health:

1. **High Blood Pressure**: Excessive salt intake can lead to increased blood pressure levels, which is a major risk factor for heart disease, stroke, and kidney problems. Consuming too much salt causes the body to retain water, leading to fluid buildup and higher blood pressure.

2. **Weight Gain**: Foods high in sugar are often calorie-dense but nutrient-poor, leading to weight gain over time. Sugary drinks, snacks, and desserts can contribute to excess calorie consumption, leading to obesity and related health problems.

3. **Insulin Resistance**: High sugar intake can lead to insulin resistance, a condition in which cells become less responsive to the effects of insulin, the hormone responsible for regulating blood sugar levels. Insulin resistance is a key factor in the development of type 2 diabetes.

4. **Increased Risk of Chronic Diseases**: Diets high in salt and sugar are associated with an increased risk of chronic diseases such as type 2 diabetes, heart disease, stroke, and certain types of cancer. Excessive salt intake can also lead to kidney damage and osteoporosis.

5. **Poor Dental Health:** Sugar promotes the growth of harmful bacteria in the mouth, leading to tooth decay and cavities. Consuming sugary foods and drinks regularly can erode tooth enamel and contribute to gum disease.

Understanding the impact of salt and sugar on our bodies is crucial for successful weight loss and overall health. By reducing salt and sugar intake and opting for whole, nutrient-rich foods instead, individuals can support their weight loss goals and improve their overall well-being.

Here are some examples of how making dietary changes can aid in weight loss:

1. **Choosing Whole Foods:** Instead of processed and packaged foods high in salt and sugar, opt for whole foods such as fruits, vegetables, lean proteins, and whole grains. These foods are lower in calories and higher in nutrients, making them more satiating and supportive of weight loss efforts.

2. **Reading Labels**: Pay attention to nutrition labels and ingredient lists when shopping for groceries. Avoid products with added sugars, high sodium content, and

artificial additives. Choose products with minimal processing and recognizable ingredients.

3. **Limiting Sugary Beverages**: Cut back on sugary drinks such as soda, fruit juice, and sweetened coffee beverages. These beverages are often high in calories and provide little to no nutritional value. Instead, opt for water, herbal tea, or unsweetened beverages.

4. **Cooking at Home:** Prepare meals at home using fresh, whole ingredients whenever possible. Cooking allows you to control the amount of salt and sugar added to your meals and enables you to make healthier choices.

5. **Mindful Eating**: Practice mindful eating by paying attention to hunger and fullness cues, savoring each bite, and eating slowly. Avoid mindless snacking and emotional eating, which can lead to overconsumption of high-calorie, high-sugar foods.

By making these dietary changes and understanding the impact of salt and sugar on our bodies, individuals can support their weight loss goals and improve their overall health and well-being.

Chapter 6: Diving into Diets: Finding What Works

In a normal American city filled with people from all walks of life, there lived two individuals who found themselves on a journey of self-discovery and transformation. Meet Emily and Michael, two average individuals who, like many others, struggled with their weight and overall health. However, with determination and perseverance, they each embarked on a path to better health through dietary changes.

Emily was a 35-year-old woman who had battled with her weight for most of her adult life. She found herself stuck in a cycle of yo-yo dieting and emotional eating, constantly searching for the next quick fix to shed pounds. But despite her efforts, she always seemed to end up right back where she started – feeling defeated and frustrated.

One day, Emily decided that enough was enough. She realized that she needed to make a permanent lifestyle change if she wanted to achieve lasting results. She began by educating herself about nutrition and experimenting with different dietary approaches to find what worked best for her body.

After much trial and error, Emily discovered that a balanced diet rich in whole foods – such as fruits, vegetables, lean proteins, and whole grains – was the key to her success. She learned to listen to her body's hunger and fullness cues, practicing mindful eating and savoring each bite.

With her newfound knowledge and determination, Emily began to see results. She lost weight steadily and felt more energetic and vibrant than ever before. But perhaps most importantly, she developed a healthier relationship with food and her body, no longer relying on diets or restriction to achieve her goals.

Meanwhile, across town, Michael was facing his own struggles with weight and health. At 40 years old, he found himself overweight and out of shape, plagued by low energy levels and frequent health issues. He knew that he needed to make a change, but he wasn't sure where to start.

After consulting with a nutritionist and doing some research of his own, Michael decided to overhaul his diet and lifestyle. He began by cutting out processed foods, sugary snacks, and fast food, replacing them with nutrient-rich whole foods.

Michael also started incorporating more plant-based meals into his diet, focusing on fruits, vegetables, legumes, and whole grains. He discovered a newfound love for cooking and experimenting with new recipes, finding joy in nourishing his body with wholesome, homemade meals.

As he made these dietary changes, Michael began to notice a dramatic improvement in his health and well-being. He lost weight steadily, his energy levels soared, and his overall mood and outlook on life improved significantly.

But perhaps the most remarkable change of all was the impact on Michael's confidence and self-esteem. As he took control of his health and transformed his body from the inside out, he felt a newfound sense of pride and empowerment. He realized that he had the power to change his life for the better, one meal at a time.

Through their journeys, Emily and Michael discovered that finding what works when it comes to diet and nutrition is not about following the latest fad or trend – it's about listening to your body, making informed choices, and finding a sustainable approach that aligns with your goals and values. And as they continued on their paths to better health, they knew that the possibilities were endless.

With each healthy meal and positive choice they made, they were one step closer to living their happiest, healthiest lives.

Exploring Dietary Diversity: A Holistic Approach to Health and Wellness

In today's world, the term "diet" has become synonymous with restrictive eating plans and quick-fix solutions for weight loss. However, true dietary success lies not in adhering to a one-size-fits-all approach, but in understanding the wide variety of diets available and finding what works best for your individual needs and preferences. Let's dive into the world of diets and explore the benefits of various dietary approaches, along with examples of meals or foods commonly associated with each diet.

Mediterranean Diet:

- **Benefits:** The Mediterranean diet is inspired by the traditional eating patterns of countries bordering the Mediterranean Sea. It emphasizes whole, minimally processed foods such as fruits, vegetables, whole grains, legumes, nuts, seeds, olive oil, and fish. This diet is rich in antioxidants, healthy fats, and fiber, and has been associated with numerous health benefits, including improved heart health, reduced risk of chronic diseases, and weight management.

- **Example Meal**: Grilled salmon with a side of quinoa salad (mixed with tomatoes, cucumbers, olives, and feta cheese) and steamed broccoli drizzled with olive oil.

Plant-Based Diet:

- **Benefits:** A plant-based diet focuses on consuming primarily foods derived from plants, such as fruits, vegetables, whole grains, legumes, nuts, and seeds. This diet is naturally high in fiber, vitamins, minerals, and antioxidants, and has been linked to lower rates of heart disease, certain cancers, and type 2 diabetes. It may also support weight management and overall well-being.

- **Example Meal**: Lentil and vegetable stir-fry served over brown rice, accompanied by a mixed green salad with avocado, nuts, and balsamic vinaigrette dressing.

Low-Carb/Keto Diet:

- **Benefits:** Low-carb and ketogenic diets restrict carbohydrate intake while increasing fat consumption, leading the body to enter a state of ketosis, where it burns fat for fuel. These diets have been shown to promote weight loss, improve blood sugar control, and increase levels of HDL (good) cholesterol. They may also reduce risk factors for heart disease and metabolic syndrome.

- **Example Meal**: Grilled chicken breast with roasted asparagus and mashed cauliflower (prepared with butter and garlic) as a low-carb alternative to mashed potatoes.

Paleo Diet:

- **Benefits:** The Paleo diet is based on the premise of eating foods similar to those consumed by our Paleolithic ancestors, such as lean meats, fish, fruits, vegetables, nuts, and seeds, while avoiding processed foods, grains, dairy, and legumes. It emphasizes whole, nutrient-dense foods and may lead to weight loss, improved blood sugar control, and reduced inflammation.

- **Example Meal**: Baked salmon with roasted sweet potatoes and a side of steamed broccoli, followed by fresh berries for dessert.

Intermittent Fasting:

- **Benefits:** Intermittent fasting involves cycling between periods of eating and fasting, with various fasting protocols available (e.g., 16/8, 5:2, alternate-day fasting). This approach may promote weight loss, improve metabolic health, and increase longevity by enhancing cellular repair processes and promoting autophagy. It may also simplify meal planning and reduce overall calorie intake.

- **Example Meal**: During the eating window, a meal might include a spinach salad with grilled chicken, avocado, and olive oil dressing, followed by Greek yogurt with berries and a handful of almonds.

While understanding and choosing the right diet is an essential component of achieving health and wellness goals, it's important to recognize that being on a diet alone is not enough to truly transform. Sustainable dietary changes must be accompanied by other lifestyle modifications, including regular physical activity, stress management, adequate sleep, and mindful eating habits.

Incorporating regular exercise into your routine helps support weight loss, improve cardiovascular health, and boost mood and energy levels. Engaging in stress-reduction techniques such as meditation, deep breathing exercises, or yoga can help reduce stress-related eating and promote overall well-being. Prioritizing quality sleep is crucial for regulating hunger hormones, supporting metabolism, and enhancing recovery and repair processes.

Additionally, practicing mindful eating involves paying attention to hunger and fullness cues, savoring each bite, and cultivating a positive relationship with food. This approach encourages enjoyment of meals without guilt or restriction, leading to greater satisfaction and long-term adherence to healthy eating habits.

By combining the right dietary approach with holistic lifestyle changes, individuals can achieve sustainable transformations that encompass both physical and mental well-being. It's not about following a strict diet for a temporary fix, but rather adopting a balanced and individualized approach that supports long-term health and vitality.

Chapter 7: Keto Kickstart: Embracing Ketogenic Eating

In a typical suburban neighborhood, there lived a woman named Rachel. Rachel had struggled with her weight and health for most of her adult life. She had tried countless diets and weight loss programs, but nothing seemed to work for her. She felt defeated and frustrated, unsure of where to turn next.

One day, while browsing the internet for solutions to her health struggles, Rachel stumbled upon the ketogenic diet. Intrigued by the promises of rapid weight loss and improved health, she decided to do some research to learn more.

As Rachel delved deeper into the science behind the ketogenic diet, she discovered that it was a low-carbohydrate, high-fat eating plan designed to shift the body into a state of ketosis, where it burns fat for fuel instead of carbohydrates. This metabolic state can lead to rapid weight loss, reduced hunger and cravings, and improved energy levels.

Inspired by the success stories she read online and the promising research behind the ketogenic diet, Rachel decided to give it a try.

She cleared her pantry of high-carb foods and stocked up on keto-friendly ingredients like avocados, nuts, seeds, olive oil, and fatty cuts of meat.

At first, Rachel found the transition to a ketogenic lifestyle challenging. She missed her favorite carb-heavy foods like bread, pasta, and sweets, and experienced some initial side effects such as fatigue and brain fog as her body adapted to burning fat for fuel. But she persisted, knowing that the potential benefits were worth it.

As Rachel continued to follow the ketogenic diet, she began to notice dramatic changes in her health and well-being. She lost weight steadily, shedding excess pounds without feeling hungry or deprived. Her energy levels soared, and she no longer experienced the energy crashes and afternoon slumps she had grown accustomed to.

But perhaps the most remarkable change of all was the improvement in Rachel's overall health. She noticed that her blood sugar levels stabilized, reducing her risk of developing type 2 diabetes. Her cholesterol levels improved, lowering her risk of heart disease. She even experienced relief from chronic inflammation and joint pain that had plagued her for years.

Inspired by Rachel's success, her friend Andrea decided to give the ketogenic diet a try as well. Andrea had struggled with her weight and health for most of her life, and traditional diets had never worked for her. But after seeing Rachel's transformation firsthand, she felt hopeful that the ketogenic diet might finally offer her a solution.

Like Rachel, Andrea experienced significant improvements in her health and well-being after adopting the ketogenic diet. She lost weight effortlessly, her energy levels skyrocketed, and she felt more confident and vibrant than ever before. She even noticed improvements in her mental clarity and focus, allowing her to be more productive and engaged in her daily life.

Through their experiences, Rachel and Andrea discovered that the ketogenic diet was more than just a weight loss plan – it was a powerful tool for transforming their health and reclaiming their lives. By embracing a low-carb, high-fat eating approach, they were able to achieve results that had eluded them for years, gaining not only physical health but also renewed vitality and happiness.

Unlocking the Power of the Keto Diet: Transformative Health and Wellness

The ketogenic diet, often referred to as the keto diet, is a high-fat, low-carbohydrate eating plan designed to shift the body into a metabolic state called ketosis. In ketosis, the body burns fat for fuel instead of carbohydrates, leading to a variety of health benefits, including weight loss, improved blood sugar control, and increased energy levels. Here's a detailed plan and explanation of a typical keto diet:

Overview of the Keto Diet:

Macronutrient Ratios:

- The keto diet typically consists of macronutrient ratios that are high in fat, moderate in protein, and very low in carbohydrates. A common macronutrient breakdown is:
  - 70-75% of calories from fat
  - 20-25% of calories from protein
  - 5-10% of calories from carbohydrates

Foods to Eat:

- Healthy fats: Avocado, olive oil, coconut oil, butter, ghee, fatty cuts of meat, fatty fish (salmon, mackerel, sardines), nuts, seeds

- Protein sources: Chicken, turkey, beef, pork, eggs, fish, tofu, tempeh

- Low-carb vegetables: Leafy greens (spinach, kale, lettuce), cruciferous vegetables (broccoli, cauliflower, cabbage), zucchini, bell peppers, avocado

- Dairy (in moderation): Full-fat cheese, cream, Greek yogurt

- Condiments and seasonings: Herbs, spices, vinegar, mustard, low-carb sauces (sugar-free BBQ sauce, hot sauce)

Foods to Avoid:

- High-carb foods: Bread, pasta, rice, grains, cereal, potatoes, sugary snacks, sweets, sugary beverages, fruits (except for small portions of berries)

- Processed foods: Chips, crackers, cookies, pastries, fast food, processed meats (sausage, bacon with added sugar)

- High-sugar condiments and sauces: Ketchup, barbecue sauce, sweetened salad dressings

Hydration:

- Drink plenty of water throughout the day to stay hydrated, especially since the keto diet can have a diuretic effect.
- Consider adding electrolytes to your water or consuming bone broth to replenish electrolytes lost through increased urination.

Typical Meal Plan:

- Breakfast: Scrambled eggs cooked in butter with spinach and cheese, topped with avocado slices.
- Lunch: Grilled chicken Caesar salad with romaine lettuce, cherry tomatoes, Parmesan cheese, and Caesar dressing made with olive oil and anchovies.
- Dinner: Baked salmon with asparagus spears roasted in olive oil and garlic butter.
- Snacks: Handful of mixed nuts, celery sticks with almond butter, cheese slices.

Duration to See Results:

The time it takes to see results on the keto diet can vary depending on individual factors such as metabolic rate, starting weight, activity level, and adherence to the diet. However, many people experience initial weight loss and increased energy levels within the first few weeks of starting the keto diet. It's not uncommon to see significant changes in body composition, including reduced body fat and increased muscle mass, within the first month of following the diet consistently.

Health Benefits of the Keto Diet:

1. **Weight Loss:** By reducing carbohydrate intake and increasing fat consumption, the keto diet can promote rapid weight loss, especially in the form of body fat. This is primarily due to the body's increased reliance on stored fat for fuel in ketosis.
2. **Improved Blood Sugar Control:** The keto diet may help stabilize blood sugar levels and improve insulin sensitivity, making it beneficial for individuals with type 2 diabetes or insulin resistance.
3. **Increased Energy Levels:** Many people report experiencing sustained energy levels and improved mental

clarity and focus on the keto diet, as ketones provide a steady source of fuel for the brain and body.

4. **Reduced Inflammation:** Some research suggests that the keto diet may have anti-inflammatory effects, which could benefit individuals with inflammatory conditions such as arthritis or autoimmune diseases.

5. **Neurological Benefits:** The keto diet has been used for decades to treat epilepsy, particularly in children who are resistant to traditional medications. It may also have potential benefits for other neurological conditions such as Alzheimer's disease and Parkinson's disease.

6. **Heart Health:** While the keto diet is high in saturated fat, it may improve certain risk factors for heart disease, such as blood triglyceride levels, HDL cholesterol levels, and blood pressure.

It's important to note that the keto diet may not be suitable for everyone, and individuals with certain medical conditions or dietary restrictions should consult with a healthcare provider before starting the diet. Additionally, long-term adherence to the keto diet may require careful planning and monitoring to ensure adequate nutrient intake and overall health.

Understanding The Potential Risks of A Strict Diets Like Keto

While the ketogenic diet can offer numerous health benefits for many individuals, it's important to be aware of potential risks and side effects associated with this eating plan. Here are some risks and considerations to keep in mind when following a keto diet:

1. **Nutrient Deficiencies**: Because the keto diet restricts certain food groups such as fruits, grains, and legumes, there is a risk of nutrient deficiencies if not carefully planned. Key nutrients that may be lacking include fiber, vitamins (especially vitamin C and B vitamins), minerals (such as magnesium and potassium), and antioxidants.

2. **Keto Flu:** When transitioning to a ketogenic diet, some people experience what is commonly known as the "keto flu," which includes symptoms such as fatigue, headache, dizziness, nausea, irritability, and difficulty concentrating. These symptoms are usually temporary and can be mitigated by staying hydrated, consuming electrolytes, and gradually reducing carbohydrate intake.

3. **Electrolyte Imbalance:** The keto diet can have a diuretic effect, leading to increased excretion of electrolytes such as sodium, potassium, and magnesium. This can result in

electrolyte imbalances, which may cause symptoms like muscle cramps, weakness, dizziness, and irregular heart rhythm. It's important to replenish electrolytes through food sources or supplements, especially during the initial stages of the diet.

4. **Gastrointestinal Issues:** Some people may experience digestive discomfort, constipation, or diarrhea when first starting the keto diet, particularly if they're not consuming enough fiber-rich foods. Gradually increasing fiber intake from low-carb vegetables, nuts, seeds, and low-carb fruits can help alleviate these symptoms.

5. **Increased Risk of Kidney Stones**: The high intake of animal proteins and fats on the keto diet may increase the risk of developing kidney stones, particularly in individuals with a history of kidney stones or kidney problems. Staying well-hydrated and consuming adequate fluids can help reduce this risk.

6. **Cholesterol Levels:** While the keto diet may improve certain lipid markers such as triglycerides and HDL cholesterol, it can also raise LDL cholesterol levels in some individuals, particularly if they're consuming large amounts of saturated fats. It's essential to monitor cholesterol levels

regularly and consult with a healthcare provider if there are concerns.

7. **Potential Long-Term Health Effects:** The long-term safety and efficacy of the ketogenic diet beyond a few years are not well-established, especially in terms of cardiovascular health and overall mortality. More research is needed to understand the potential risks and benefits of sustained ketosis over extended periods.

8. **Adherence and Social Impact:** The strict dietary restrictions of the keto diet may be challenging for some individuals to maintain long-term, especially in social situations or when dining out. It's essential to consider the practicality and sustainability of the diet for your lifestyle and personal preferences.

Overall, while the ketogenic diet can be effective for weight loss and certain health conditions, it's essential to approach it with caution and consult with a healthcare provider or registered dietitian before making significant dietary changes, especially if you have underlying health conditions or concerns. A personalized approach that considers individual health goals, preferences, and medical history is key to maximizing the potential benefits of the keto diet while minimizing risks.

Chapter 8: The Power of Caloric Deficit: Eating for Weight Loss

Meet Alex, a 32-year-old marketing executive who had struggled with his weight for years. Despite trying various diets and exercise programs, he always found himself back at square one, feeling frustrated and defeated. It wasn't until he learned about the concept of a caloric deficit that everything changed.

Alex stumbled upon the idea of a caloric deficit while researching different weight loss strategies online. Intrigued by the science behind it, he decided to give it a try. A caloric deficit is achieved by consuming fewer calories than the body expends, leading to weight loss over time. It's a simple concept, but one that Alex had never fully understood or implemented before.

Armed with this newfound knowledge, Alex set out to create a plan that would put him in a caloric deficit while still providing his body with the nutrients it needed to thrive. He started by calculating his basal metabolic rate (BMR) and total daily energy expenditure (TDEE) using online calculators, which gave him an estimate of how many calories he needed to maintain his current weight.

Next, Alex decided to reduce his daily calorie intake by 500-750 calories below his TDEE, a moderate deficit that would allow for steady, sustainable weight loss. He focused on making small, gradual changes to his diet, such as reducing portion sizes, cutting back on sugary snacks and beverages, and incorporating more whole, nutrient-dense foods like fruits, vegetables, lean proteins, and whole grains.

In addition to adjusting his diet, Alex also started incorporating regular exercise into his routine to further increase his calorie deficit and improve his overall health. He began with simple activities like walking, jogging, and cycling, gradually increasing the intensity and duration of his workouts as he built strength and endurance.

As the weeks passed, Alex began to see noticeable changes in his body and overall well-being. He lost weight steadily, dropping pounds week after week as he continued to adhere to his caloric deficit plan. He felt more energetic and confident than ever before, enjoying newfound freedom and flexibility in his dietary choices while still making progress toward his weight loss goals.

By the end of six months, Alex had lost a total of 50 pounds, an achievement he never thought possible. But perhaps even more importantly, he had gained a deeper understanding of his body and how to nourish it properly. The concept of a caloric deficit had empowered him to take control of his health and transform his life for the better.

Alex's success story is not unique. Research has shown that creating a caloric deficit through diet and exercise is one of the most effective ways to achieve sustainable weight loss over time. By understanding the science behind weight loss and implementing practical strategies like calorie tracking and portion control, anyone can achieve their weight loss goals and improve their overall health and well-being.

Understanding Caloric Deficit:

Let's break down the concept of caloric deficit and how it can be harnessed as a powerful tool for weight loss, along with a plan to implement it effectively:

What is Caloric Deficit?

Caloric deficit simply means consuming fewer calories than your body expends. When you consistently maintain a caloric deficit over time, your body will tap into stored fat for energy, leading to weight loss.

How Does it Work?

Your body requires a certain amount of energy (calories) to maintain its current weight, known as Total Daily Energy Expenditure (TDEE). By consuming fewer calories than your TDEE, you create a deficit, prompting your body to use stored fat for fuel.

Calculating Your Caloric Needs:

1. **Basal Metabolic Rate (BMR)**: This is the number of calories your body needs to maintain basic physiological functions at rest. You can use an online calculator to estimate your BMR based on factors like age, gender, weight, and height.
2. **Total Daily Energy Expenditure (TDEE):** This is your BMR multiplied by an activity factor that represents your

daily activity level. Again, online calculators can provide an estimate based on your activity level.

3. **Creating a Deficit:** To lose weight, aim to consume 500-750 calories less than your TDEE per day. This typically results in a safe and sustainable weight loss of 1-2 pounds per week.

Advantages of Caloric Deficit:

1. **Effective Weight Loss**: Caloric deficit is one of the most effective methods for losing weight, as it directly addresses the energy balance equation.
2. **Flexibility:** Unlike restrictive diets, caloric deficit allows for flexibility in food choices, as long as overall calorie intake is controlled.
3. **Sustainable:** By focusing on gradual, sustainable changes to your eating habits, caloric deficit can lead to long-term success.
4. **Preserves Lean Muscle**: When combined with adequate protein intake and resistance training, caloric deficit can help preserve lean muscle mass while losing fat.

Difficulties and Challenges:

1. **Initial Adjustment:** Adjusting to a lower calorie intake may be challenging at first, as your body adapts to the new energy balance.

2. **Hunger and Cravings:** You may experience increased hunger and cravings, especially if you're used to eating larger portions or calorie-dense foods.

3. **Social Pressures**: Social situations and peer pressure can make it difficult to adhere to your calorie goals, especially when dining out or attending social events.

4. **Plateaus**: Weight loss may plateau over time as your body adjusts to the lower calorie intake, requiring adjustments to your diet or exercise routine.

Implementing a Caloric Deficit Plan:

1. **Track Your Intake**: Use a food diary or mobile app to track your daily calorie intake, aiming to stay within your prescribed deficit.

2. **Prioritize Nutrient-Dense Foods:** Focus on filling your diet with nutrient-dense foods like fruits, vegetables, lean proteins, and whole grains to maximize satiety and meet your nutritional needs.

3. **Practice Portion Control:** Be mindful of portion sizes and avoid mindless eating, especially when dining out or snacking.

4. **Incorporate Exercise:** While not strictly necessary for weight loss, regular exercise can enhance the calorie deficit and improve overall health.

5. **Stay Consistent:** Consistency is key to success with caloric deficit. Stick to your plan even on days when motivation is low, and remember that progress takes time.

Caloric deficit is a powerful and scientifically proven approach to weight loss that can be customized to fit your individual needs and preferences. By understanding the principles of energy balance and implementing practical strategies like tracking your intake, prioritizing nutrient-dense foods, and staying consistent, you can achieve your weight loss goals and improve your overall health and well-being. Remember, small changes add up over time, so stay patient and trust the process!

Chapter 9: Mindful Eating: Being Present at the Table

In a busy city, amidst the chaos of daily life, there lived a young woman named Maya. Maya was always on the go, juggling work deadlines, social commitments, and family responsibilities. In the midst of her hectic schedule, she often found herself rushing through meals, barely pausing to taste or enjoy the food on her plate.

One day, after yet another stressful day at the office, Maya decided to make a change. She realized that she had been neglecting her health and well-being by mindlessly eating on the go, and she longed to reconnect with the joy of nourishing her body with wholesome food.

Maya began to explore the concept of mindful eating – the practice of being fully present and aware while eating, paying attention to the sensory experience of food and the signals of hunger and satiety from the body. She learned that mindful eating isn't just about what we eat, but also about how we eat and the mindset we bring to the table.

With newfound determination, Maya set out to cultivate a more mindful approach to eating. She started by carving out dedicated time for meals, free from distractions like smartphones or television. She set the table with care, lighting a candle and taking a moment to express gratitude for the nourishment before her.

As Maya sat down to eat, she focused on savoring each bite, noticing the colors, textures, and flavors of the food. She took her time chewing slowly and thoroughly, allowing her body to fully digest and absorb the nutrients. With each mindful bite, she felt a sense of calm and contentment wash over her, as if she were truly nourishing her body and soul from within.

Over time, Maya began to notice profound changes in her relationship with food and her overall well-being. She found that she no longer craved unhealthy snacks or overindulged in emotional eating. Instead, she listened to her body's cues of hunger and satiety, eating when she was hungry and stopping when she was full.

As Maya continued to practice mindful eating, she also discovered a newfound appreciation for the connection between food and mental health. She realized that nourishing her body with wholesome, nutrient-rich foods not only supported physical vitality but also enhanced her mood and cognitive function.

With each mindful meal, Maya felt more grounded, centered, and present in her own life. She embraced the simple pleasure of sharing nourishing food with loved ones, fostering deeper connections and moments of joy around the dinner table.

Through her journey of mindful eating, Maya learned that true nourishment extends beyond the food on our plates – it's about cultivating a deeper awareness and appreciation for the abundance of life's simple pleasures. And as she savored each mindful bite, she found fulfillment and nourishment in both body and soul.

Mindful eating, also known as mindful nutrition or mindful consumption, is the practice of cultivating awareness and presence while eating. It involves paying full attention to the sensory experience of food, as well as to the thoughts, emotions, and physical sensations that arise before, during, and after eating. The goal of mindful eating is to develop a more conscious and intentional relationship with food, leading to improved overall health and well-being.

Here's how mindful eating works and how it benefits our health:

1. Awareness of Hunger and Satiety Signals:

Mindful eating encourages individuals to tune into their body's hunger and satiety cues. By paying attention to physical sensations such as stomach growling, feelings of fullness, and satisfaction after a meal, people can better regulate their food intake and avoid overeating.

2. Enhanced Sensory Experience:

When practicing mindful eating, individuals focus on the sensory qualities of food, including its appearance, aroma, taste, and texture. By fully engaging the senses, people can derive greater enjoyment and satisfaction from their meals, leading to a more pleasurable eating experience.

3. Prevention of Emotional Eating:

Mindful eating helps individuals become more attuned to their emotional triggers for eating, such as stress, boredom, or sadness. By cultivating awareness of these triggers, people can develop healthier coping mechanisms and make more conscious choices about when, what, and how much they eat.

4. Improved Digestion:

Eating mindfully involves chewing food slowly and thoroughly, which aids in the digestive process. Proper chewing allows for better breakdown of food particles, leading to improved nutrient absorption and reduced risk of digestive discomfort such as bloating, gas, and indigestion.

5. Reduction of Food-Related Stress:

Mindful eating encourages individuals to approach food with a non-judgmental and compassionate attitude. By letting go of restrictive diet rules and guilt-inducing thoughts about food, people can reduce stress and anxiety related to eating, leading to a more positive and relaxed relationship with food.

6. Weight Management:

Studies have shown that mindful eating practices can contribute to weight management and weight loss. By increasing awareness of portion sizes, eating patterns, and food choices, individuals are better equipped to make healthier decisions and maintain a balanced diet.

7. Promotion of Healthy Eating Habits:

Over time, practicing mindful eating can lead to the development of healthier eating habits. By being more mindful of food choices, individuals may naturally gravitate towards nourishing, whole foods that support their overall health and well-being.

In summary, mindful eating involves bringing a non-judgmental, present-focused awareness to the act of eating, leading to a more positive and balanced relationship with food and improved health outcomes.

Cultivating Presence and Awareness at the Table

Here are some examples of mindful eating practices that can help cultivate presence and awareness at the table:

1. **Engage Your Senses:** Take a moment to notice the colors, textures, and aromas of your food before taking a bite. Notice the vibrant hues of fruits and vegetables, the

fragrant aroma of herbs and spices, and the satisfying crunch of fresh greens.

2. **Chew Slowly and Thoroughly**: Instead of rushing through your meal, take the time to chew each bite slowly and thoroughly. Pay attention to the sensation of food in your mouth, and notice how the flavors and textures evolve with each chew.

3. **Savor Each Bite:** As you eat, focus on savoring the taste and texture of each bite. Notice the subtle nuances of flavor – the sweetness of ripe fruit, the earthiness of whole grains, or the richness of creamy dairy. Take pleasure in the sensory experience of eating.

4. **Listen to Your Body:** Tune into your body's hunger and fullness signals as you eat. Eat when you're hungry and stop when you're comfortably satisfied, rather than eating out of habit or boredom. Trust your body to guide you in making nourishing choices.

5. **Minimize Distractions:** Create a peaceful and distraction-free environment for your meals. Turn off the television, put away your phone, and focus solely on the act of eating. Eating without distractions allows you to fully savor the experience and tune into your body's cues.

6. **Express Gratitude**: Before you begin eating, take a moment to express gratitude for the food in front of you. Acknowledge the effort that went into growing, preparing, and serving the meal, and cultivate a sense of appreciation for the nourishment it provides.

7. **Practice Mindful Portion Control:** Pay attention to portion sizes and serve yourself appropriate portions based on your hunger and energy needs. Avoid mindless overeating by checking in with your body's hunger and fullness signals throughout the meal.

8. **Notice Emotional Triggers:** Be mindful of emotional eating triggers, such as stress, boredom, or sadness. Instead of turning to food as a source of comfort, explore alternative ways to cope with emotions, such as journaling, meditation, or spending time in nature.

9. **Eat with Intention:** Approach each meal with intention and purpose, choosing foods that nourish your body and support your overall health and well-being. Make conscious decisions about what you eat, and enjoy the process of nurturing yourself through food.

By incorporating these mindful eating practices into your daily routine, you can cultivate a deeper sense of presence and awareness at the table, fostering a healthier relationship with food and enhancing your overall well-being.

Chapter 10: Gender Differences in Weight Loss: Bridging the Gap

Meet Jack and Emily, two individuals on a quest to improve their health and wellness through weight loss. While their journeys may differ in some ways due to their gender, they both share a common goal: to achieve lasting health and happiness.

Jack, a 35-year-old software engineer, has struggled with his weight for years. As a man, he feels pressure to conform to societal ideals of masculinity, which often equate being fit and muscular with strength and success. However, Jack finds himself falling short of these expectations, grappling with excess weight and a sedentary lifestyle.

Emily, a 30-year-old graphic designer, also faces her own challenges when it comes to weight loss. As a woman, she feels bombarded by unrealistic beauty standards portrayed in the media, which can lead to feelings of inadequacy and self-doubt. Despite her best efforts, Emily finds it difficult to prioritize her health amidst the demands of work and family life.

Despite their differences, Jack and Emily both recognize the importance of taking control of their health and making positive changes. They decide to embark on their weight loss journeys together, supporting and encouraging each other every step of the way.

As they delve into the world of nutrition and fitness, Jack and Emily discover that there are indeed some differences between how men and women approach weight loss. For example, men typically have a higher basal metabolic rate (BMR) and tend to lose weight more quickly than women due to differences in body composition and hormone levels.

However, Jack and Emily also learn that these differences don't have to hold them back. By understanding their unique needs and challenges, they can tailor their approach to weight loss to fit their individual lifestyles and preferences.

For Jack, this might mean focusing on building muscle through strength training exercises, which can help boost his metabolism and burn calories more efficiently. He also learns the importance of incorporating protein-rich foods into his diet to support muscle growth and repair.

Meanwhile, Emily discovers the benefits of high-intensity interval training (HIIT) and circuit training workouts, which are particularly effective for burning fat and improving cardiovascular health. She also learns to prioritize self-care and stress management techniques, such as meditation and yoga, to support her overall well-being.

Despite the occasional setbacks and challenges they encounter along the way, Jack and Emily remain committed to their goals. They celebrate each other's successes, whether it's hitting a new personal best at the gym or resisting the temptation to indulge in unhealthy foods.

As their weight loss journeys progress, Jack and Emily both experience significant improvements in their health and happiness. They feel more confident and empowered, knowing that they have the knowledge and tools to take control of their bodies and their lives.

In the end, Jack and Emily prove that with the right knowledge, effort, and support, anyone can achieve their weight loss goals and live a healthy, happy life, regardless of their gender. They serve as inspiration to others, showing that true strength comes from within, and that by working together, we can overcome any obstacle that stands in our way.

When it comes to weight loss, both men and women may encounter unique challenges based on their gender, body composition, hormonal differences, and societal expectations. Understanding these differences and implementing strategies tailored to individual needs can help both genders achieve their weight loss goals and stay motivated throughout their journey.

Challenges for Men:

1. **Higher BMR and Muscle Mass:** Men typically have a higher basal metabolic rate (BMR) and greater muscle mass compared to women, which means they tend to burn more calories at rest. However, this can also lead to higher

calorie requirements and potentially greater hunger levels, making it challenging to maintain a caloric deficit.

2. **Pressure to Build Muscle**: Many men feel pressure to achieve a muscular physique, which may lead to a focus on muscle-building exercises rather than prioritizing overall health and weight loss. This emphasis on strength training alone may neglect other important aspects of fitness, such as cardiovascular health and flexibility.

Solutions for Men:

1. **Balanced Approach to Exercise:** While strength training is important for building muscle and boosting metabolism, men should also incorporate cardiovascular exercise and flexibility training into their routines. This helps to improve overall fitness and support weight loss by burning calories and enhancing metabolic health.

2. **Mindful Eating Habits**: Men can benefit from adopting mindful eating practices to better regulate hunger and satiety cues. This involves paying attention to portion sizes, eating slowly, and choosing nutrient-dense foods that support overall health and weight management.

Challenges for Women:

1. **Lower BMR and Hormonal Fluctuations**: Women tend to have a lower BMR and less muscle mass compared to men, which means they typically burn fewer calories at rest. Additionally, hormonal fluctuations throughout the menstrual cycle can affect appetite, energy levels, and metabolism, making weight loss more challenging.

2. **Body Image and Societal Pressures**: Women may face intense societal pressure to achieve an unrealistic standard of beauty, leading to feelings of inadequacy and self-doubt. This can contribute to disordered eating patterns, emotional eating, and difficulty maintaining a healthy relationship with food.

Solutions for Women:

1. **Hormonal Awareness:** Women can benefit from understanding how hormonal fluctuations affect appetite and metabolism throughout the menstrual cycle. By tracking their cycle and adjusting their nutrition and exercise routines accordingly, women can better manage energy levels and cravings.

2. **Focus on Strength and Empowerment:** Instead of striving for an unattainable ideal of thinness, women can shift their focus towards strength, empowerment, and overall health. Strength training can help women build lean muscle mass, boost metabolism, and improve body composition, leading to increased confidence and self-esteem.

General Strategies for Both Genders:

1. **Balanced Nutrition:** Both men and women should focus on consuming a balanced diet rich in whole, nutrient-dense foods such as fruits, vegetables, lean proteins, whole grains, and healthy fats. This provides essential nutrients for optimal health and supports weight loss by promoting satiety and stabilizing blood sugar levels.

2. **Regular Exercise:** Incorporating regular physical activity into daily life is essential for both men and women to support weight loss and overall health. This includes a combination of cardiovascular exercise, strength training, and flexibility training to improve fitness, burn calories, and enhance metabolic health.

3. **Mindfulness and Self-Compassion:** Both genders can benefit from practicing mindfulness and self-compassion when it comes to weight loss. This involves being present and aware of thoughts, feelings, and behaviors related to food and body image, and cultivating a non-judgmental and compassionate attitude towards oneself.

By recognizing and addressing the unique challenges and needs of each gender, individuals can overcome obstacles to weight loss and achieve their health and wellness goals. With patience, perseverance, and support, both men and women can navigate their weight loss journey with confidence and success.

Chapter 11: Hormones and Weight: Balancing the Equation

In the small city of Brooksville, two individuals found themselves on parallel paths, each grappling with their own hormonal struggles on their weight loss journey. Meet Julia and Mark, both determined to overcome their challenges and reclaim their health and happiness.

Julia, a 38-year-old marketing manager, had long struggled with hormonal imbalances that seemed to thwart her weight loss efforts at every turn. Despite her best efforts to eat healthily and exercise regularly, she found herself constantly battling cravings, mood swings, and stubborn weight gain.

Meanwhile, Mark, a 42-year-old accountant, faced his own hormonal hurdles on his weight loss journey. Years of stress and unhealthy lifestyle habits had taken a toll on his hormonal health, leaving him feeling exhausted, irritable, and frustrated with his lack of progress.

Despite their struggles, Julia and Mark refused to give up hope. They both sought guidance from a holistic health coach who specialized in hormonal imbalances and weight loss. With the coach's support and expertise, Julia and Mark embarked on a journey of healing and transformation.

Together, they delved into the root causes of their hormonal imbalances, exploring factors such as stress, sleep, diet, and environmental toxins. Through targeted testing and personalized nutrition plans, they began to address imbalances in key hormones such as cortisol, insulin, thyroid, and sex hormones.

For Julia, this meant focusing on stress management techniques such as meditation, yoga, and deep breathing exercises to lower cortisol levels and support adrenal health. She also implemented dietary changes to stabilize blood sugar levels and support healthy hormone production.

Meanwhile, Mark focused on optimizing his sleep hygiene and reducing exposure to endocrine-disrupting chemicals found in plastics, pesticides, and personal care products. He also incorporated specific foods and supplements known to support testosterone production and balance estrogen levels.

As they progressed on their journey, both Julia and Mark began to notice profound changes in their health and well-being. Julia's cravings diminished, her energy levels soared, and she shed excess weight effortlessly. Mark's mood stabilized, his energy returned, and he started to see improvements in his body composition and muscle tone.

Their success didn't come overnight, and there were certainly bumps along the way. But with patience, perseverance, and the support of their coach, Julia and Mark overcame their hormonal hurdles and emerged stronger and healthier than ever before.

Their journey serves as a testament to the power of addressing hormonal imbalances in weight loss and the importance of taking a holistic approach to health and wellness. By understanding their bodies' unique needs and supporting hormonal balance through lifestyle changes, Julia and Mark reclaimed control of their health and transformed their lives for the better.

Understanding How Hormones Can Impact Our Health

Any personal trainer or health professional can attest, it's important to understand that hormonal imbalances can significantly impact weight loss efforts. Here's a beginner-friendly explanation of different hormone issues and strategies to overcome them:

Hormone Issues Affecting Weight Loss:

1. **Insulin Resistance**: Insulin is a hormone that regulates blood sugar levels. Insulin resistance occurs when cells become less responsive to insulin, leading to elevated blood sugar levels and increased fat storage, especially around the abdomen.

2. **Cortisol Imbalance:** Cortisol is known as the stress hormone and plays a role in metabolism, inflammation, and

fat storage. Chronic stress can lead to elevated cortisol levels, which may increase appetite, promote fat storage, and hinder weight loss efforts.

3. **Thyroid Dysfunction:** The thyroid gland produces hormones that regulate metabolism and energy production. Hypothyroidism (underactive thyroid) can lead to a sluggish metabolism and weight gain, while hyperthyroidism (overactive thyroid) can cause weight loss despite increased appetite.

4. **Sex Hormone Imbalance**: Hormones such as estrogen, progesterone, and testosterone play a role in regulating metabolism, fat distribution, and appetite. Imbalances in these hormones, often seen in conditions like polycystic ovary syndrome (PCOS) or andropause, can contribute to weight gain and difficulty losing weight.

Strategies to Overcome Hormonal Imbalances:

1. **Balanced Nutrition:** Focus on a balanced diet rich in whole, nutrient-dense foods such as fruits, vegetables, lean proteins, and healthy fats. Limit processed foods, refined sugars, and excessive carbohydrates, which can exacerbate insulin resistance and hormonal imbalances.

2. **Regular Exercise:** Incorporate regular physical activity into your routine, including both cardiovascular exercise and strength training. Exercise helps regulate hormone levels, improve insulin sensitivity, and support metabolic health.

3. **Stress Management:** Practice stress-reducing techniques such as meditation, deep breathing exercises, yoga, or mindfulness practices. Managing stress levels can help lower cortisol levels and reduce the impact of chronic stress on hormonal balance.

4. **Adequate Sleep:** Prioritize quality sleep, aiming for 7-9 hours per night. Poor sleep can disrupt hormone levels, including cortisol and growth hormone, which are important for regulating metabolism and supporting weight loss.

5. **Supplementation:** Consider targeted supplements or herbs that support hormonal balance, such as omega-3 fatty acids, vitamin D, magnesium, and adaptogenic herbs like ashwagandha or rhodiola. However, always consult with a healthcare professional before starting any new supplements.

6. **Medical Evaluation:** If you suspect you have a hormonal imbalance impacting your weight loss efforts, consult with a healthcare provider or endocrinologist for evaluation and appropriate treatment options. They may recommend hormone testing, medication, or other interventions to address underlying issues.

By understanding the role of hormones in weight loss and implementing strategies to support hormonal balance, individuals can overcome obstacles and achieve their health and fitness goals more effectively. It's important to approach weight loss from a holistic perspective, addressing both lifestyle factors and underlying hormonal imbalances for long-term success.

Chapter 12: Muscles in Motion: Building Strength

Once upon a time in Oakwood, lived Alex and Mia, two individuals on a quest for better health and vitality. Both Alex, a 28-year-old software developer, and Mia, a 30-year-old teacher, had spent years leading sedentary lifestyles, plagued by poor dietary choices and lack of physical activity.

Alex had always been self-conscious about his slender frame, while Mia struggled with excess weight and low energy levels. Determined to make a change, they embarked on a journey of transformation together, armed with newfound knowledge and a shared commitment to improving their health.

Alex's Journey:

Alex began his journey by incorporating regular strength training sessions into his weekly routine. He started with basic bodyweight exercises like push-ups, squats, and lunges, gradually progressing to more challenging movements with weights and resistance bands. He focused on compound exercises that targeted multiple muscle groups simultaneously, such as deadlifts, bench presses, and rows.

In addition to strength training, Alex made significant changes to his diet, emphasizing lean proteins, complex carbohydrates, and healthy fats. He swapped out processed foods and sugary snacks for whole, nutrient-dense options like grilled chicken, brown rice, avocado, and leafy greens. He also prioritized protein-rich snacks like Greek yogurt, nuts, and protein shakes to support muscle growth and repair.

As Alex's fitness level increased and his body composition began to change, he experienced a newfound sense of confidence and strength. His muscles grew stronger and more defined, and he noticed improvements in his posture, energy levels, and overall well-being. With each workout, he felt a sense of accomplishment and empowerment, knowing that he was taking control of his health and fitness.

Mia's Journey:

Meanwhile, Mia embarked on her own journey of transformation, starting with regular cardiovascular exercise to kickstart her weight loss efforts. She began with brisk walks around her neighborhood, gradually increasing the intensity and duration of her workouts over time. She also incorporated other forms of cardio such as cycling, swimming, and dance classes to keep her workouts fun and engaging.

In addition to cardio, Mia focused on strength training to build lean muscle mass and boost her metabolism. She started with light weights and resistance bands, gradually increasing the intensity and volume of her workouts as she grew stronger. She also incorporated bodyweight exercises like squats, lunges, and planks to target different muscle groups and improve her overall strength and stability.

Diet-wise, Mia made significant changes to her eating habits, focusing on portion control, balanced meals, and mindful eating. She swapped out high-calorie, processed foods for whole, nutrient-dense options like lean proteins, colorful fruits and vegetables, and whole grains. She also paid attention to her hunger and satiety cues, eating slowly and mindfully to prevent overeating and promote better digestion.

As Mia's fitness level improved and her body began to transform, she noticed significant changes in her weight, body composition, and overall health. She shed excess pounds, toned her muscles, and gained confidence in her appearance and abilities. She felt more energized and motivated than ever before, inspired by the progress she had made and excited for the journey ahead.

Conclusion:

Through their dedication to regular exercise and a balanced diet, Alex and Mia both achieved remarkable transformations, both physically and mentally. They proved that with the right knowledge, effort, and support, anyone can overcome the challenges of a sedentary lifestyle and embark on a journey of health, happiness, and vitality. Their stories serve as inspiration to others, showing that positive change is possible, one step at a time.

The Vital Connection Between Weight Loss, Muscle Health and Logevity

In the pursuit of longevity and optimal health, two key pillars stand out: weight loss and muscle health. Both play integral roles in promoting overall well-being and longevity, and understanding their importance can empower individuals to make positive changes in their lives.

Weight loss, when achieved in a sustainable and healthy manner, offers numerous benefits beyond aesthetics. Excess body weight, especially when concentrated around vital organs, can increase the risk of chronic diseases such as heart disease, type 2 diabetes, and certain cancers. By shedding excess pounds, individuals can significantly reduce their risk of developing these conditions and improve their overall quality of life.

Furthermore, weight loss has been linked to improvements in metabolic health, including better insulin sensitivity, blood sugar control, and cholesterol levels. These metabolic changes can translate into increased energy levels, improved mood, and reduced inflammation, all of which contribute to a longer and healthier life.

Equally important is the preservation and maintenance of muscle mass. As we age, we naturally lose muscle mass and strength, a process known as sarcopenia. This decline in muscle mass not only affects physical performance but also increases the risk of falls, fractures, and loss of independence in older adults.

However, regular exercise, particularly strength training, can help counteract sarcopenia by stimulating muscle growth and improving muscle function. Building and maintaining muscle mass not only enhances physical strength and mobility but also supports metabolic health, bone density, and overall vitality as we age.

Moreover, muscle tissue is metabolically active, meaning it burns more calories at rest compared to fat tissue. By increasing muscle mass, individuals can boost their basal metabolic rate, making it easier to maintain a healthy weight and prevent weight regain.

In essence, the symbiotic relationship between weight loss and muscle health forms the foundation for longevity and optimal health. By prioritizing both aspects through lifestyle modifications such as regular exercise and a balanced diet, individuals can enhance their chances of living a longer, healthier, and more fulfilling life.

One significant statistic regarding muscle mass and longevity comes from a study published in the American Journal of Medicine, which found that individuals with higher levels of muscle mass have a lower risk of mortality. Specifically, the study found that for each 10% increase in skeletal muscle mass, there was an 11% reduction in the likelihood of death from any cause among middle-aged and older adults. This highlights the important role that muscle mass plays in promoting longevity and overall health.

In the pages that follow, we will explore actionable strategies, evidence-based practices, and practical tips to help you embark on a journey towards lasting weight loss, improved muscle health, and ultimately, a brighter and healthier future.

Here are some compound muscle exercises for each major muscle group, followed by conditioning exercises for weight loss and endurance:

Tips for Beginners:

- Start with a combination of compound muscle exercises and conditioning exercises to target all major muscle groups and improve cardiovascular health.
- Begin with lighter weights or resistance and gradually increase as you gain strength and confidence.
- Incorporate a variety of exercises to keep workouts interesting and prevent boredom or plateaus.
- Listen to your body and rest when needed. It's important to allow for adequate recovery time between workouts.
- Stay hydrated and fuel your body with nutritious foods to support energy levels and recovery.
- Consistency is key. Aim for at least 3-4 workouts per week to see progress and results over time.

Compound Muscle Exercises: Compound muscle exercises, also known as multi-joint exercises, are movements that engage multiple muscle groups and joints simultaneously. Unlike isolation exercises, which target a single muscle group and joint, compound exercises involve coordinated movements across several joints, allowing for greater muscle activation and functional strength development.

These exercises typically involve complex movements that mimic real-life activities and sports movements, making them highly effective for improving overall strength, power, and functional fitness. Examples of compound muscle exercises include squats, deadlifts, bench presses, pull-ups, and lunges. By incorporating compound exercises into a workout routine, individuals can efficiently work multiple muscle groups in less time, leading to more comprehensive muscle development and improved overall fitness.

Upper Body:

Chest:

- Bench Press (Barbell or Dumbbell)
- Push-Ups
- Chest Dips

Back:

- Deadlifts

* Pull-Ups or Lat Pull-Downs

* Bent-Over Rows (Barbell or Dumbbell)

Shoulders:

* Overhead Press (Barbell or Dumbbell)

* Arnold Press

* Lateral Raises

Lower Body:

Quadriceps:

* Squats (Barbell, Dumbbell, or Bodyweight)

* Lunges (Forward, Reverse, or Walking)

* Leg Press

Hamstrings:

* Deadlifts (Sumo or Romanian)

* Romanian Deadlifts (Barbell or Dumbbell)

* Hamstring Curls (Machine or Stability Ball)

Glutes:

* Hip Thrusts

* Bulgarian Split Squats

* Glute Bridges

Calves:

* Calf Raises (Standing or Seated)

- Donkey Calf Raises

- Jump Squats (Engaging Calf Muscles)

Core:

Abdominals:

- Planks (Front, Side, or Reverse)

- Russian Twists

- Bicycle Crunches

Conditioning Exercises for Weight Loss and Endurance:
Conditioning exercises, also known as cardiovascular or cardio exercises, are activities that elevate the heart rate and increase the body's overall endurance and cardiovascular fitness. These exercises focus on improving the efficiency of the cardiovascular system, including the heart, lungs, and blood vessels, to deliver oxygen and nutrients to working muscles more effectively.

These exercises can vary in intensity and duration, ranging from low- to high-intensity activities. Examples of conditioning exercises include running, cycling, swimming, jumping rope, and aerobic dance. These activities can be performed continuously or in intervals to challenge the cardiovascular system and enhance aerobic capacity.

In addition to improving cardiovascular health, conditioning exercises also help burn calories, promote weight loss, and boost metabolism. They can also improve mood, reduce stress, and increase energy levels, making them essential components of a well-rounded fitness program. Incorporating conditioning exercises into a regular workout routine can help individuals achieve and maintain overall health and fitness.

Cardiovascular Exercise:
- Walking or Jogging
- Cycling (Outdoor or Stationary)
- Swimming or Water Aerobics
- Rowing Machine
- Jump Rope

High-Intensity Interval Training (HIIT):
- Burpees
- Mountain Climbers
- High Knees
- Jump Squats
- Sprints (On Treadmill, Track, or Outdoor)

Circuit Training:

- Full-Body Workouts Combining Resistance and Cardio Exercises
- Circuit Machines (Rotating through different exercises with minimal rest)

Plyometric Exercises:

- Box Jumps
- Plyo Push-Ups
- Jump Lunges
- Skaters

Agility Drills:

- Ladder Drills (Forward, Lateral, or Crossover)
- Cone Drills (Shuttle Runs, Zig-Zag Runs)
- Agility Hurdles

Bodyweight Exercises:

- Squat Jumps
- Burpees
- Mountain Climbers
- Jumping Jacks

Remember, everyone's fitness journey is unique, so don't compare yourself to others. Focus on your own progress and celebrate your achievements along the way!

Chapter 13: HIIT: High-Intensity Interval Training

In the heart of Chicago, Veronica found herself at a crossroads in her fitness journey. Despite her dedication to regular gym workouts, she couldn't seem to shed the extra weight that had crept up over the years. Frustrated by the lack of results and feeling discouraged, Veronica began to question whether her efforts were in vain.

Determined to break through her plateau, Veronica decided to shake up her workout routine and explore new fitness options. After hearing rave reviews about High-Intensity Interval Training (HIIT) from friends and colleagues, she decided to give it a try, hoping that it would be the solution she had been searching for.

As Veronica stepped into the HIIT studio for her first class, she felt a mixture of excitement and apprehension. The instructor greeted her with a warm smile and explained the concept of HIIT: short bursts of intense exercise followed by brief periods of rest or low-intensity recovery. Intrigued by the promise of a more efficient and effective workout, Veronica eagerly joined the class, ready to give it her all.

The next 45 minutes flew by in a blur of sweat, determination, and adrenaline as Veronica pushed herself to her limits with a series of high-intensity exercises, including sprints, burpees, and plyometric jumps. With each interval, she felt her heart rate skyrocket and her muscles burn with exertion, but she refused to give up, fueled by a newfound sense of purpose and determination.

As the class came to an end and Veronica caught her breath, she couldn't help but feel a surge of exhilaration and accomplishment wash over her. Despite the intensity of the workout, she felt more alive and invigorated than ever before, knowing that she had pushed herself beyond her comfort zone and emerged stronger and more resilient on the other side.

In the days and weeks that followed, Veronica continued to incorporate HIIT into her fitness routine, attending classes regularly and pushing herself to new heights with each session. Slowly but surely, she began to notice changes in her body: her clothes fit more comfortably, her energy levels soared, and she felt stronger and more confident than ever before.

But perhaps most importantly, Veronica discovered a newfound sense of empowerment and self-belief that transcended the physical results. Through HIIT, she had learned to push past her limits, embrace discomfort, and embrace the power of resilience and determination. And as she stood tall, drenched in sweat and glowing with pride, Veronica knew that she had found her path to success, one high-intensity interval at a time.

What is HIIT Anyways?

High-Intensity Interval Training (HIIT) is a form of cardiovascular exercise that alternates short bursts of intense anaerobic exercise with brief periods of low-intensity recovery or rest. HIIT workouts typically involve pushing oneself to maximum effort during the high-intensity intervals, followed by periods of active recovery or rest to allow the heart rate to decrease slightly before the next interval begins. This cycle of intense exertion and recovery is repeated for a set duration, typically ranging from 10 to 30 minutes.

HIIT is known for its efficiency in burning calories, improving cardiovascular fitness, boosting metabolism, and increasing muscle strength and endurance. It can be performed using various forms of exercise, including running, cycling, rowing, bodyweight exercises, and plyometrics. HIIT workouts are popular for their time-saving benefits and ability to deliver significant fitness results in a relatively short amount of time.

Example HIIT Workouts For Begginers

Here are some examples of High-Intensity Interval Training (HIIT) workouts that you can try:

Beginner HIIT Workout:

- **Warm up:** 5 minutes of light cardio (e.g., jogging in place, jumping jacks).
- **HIIT Circuit:**
    - 30 seconds of jumping squats
    - 30 seconds of push-ups
    - 30 seconds of mountain climbers
    - 30 seconds of burpees
- **Rest:** 30 seconds
- Repeat the circuit 3-4 times.
- **Cool down:** 5 minutes of stretching.

Bodyweight HIIT Workout:

- **Warm up:** 5 minutes of dynamic stretching (e.g., arm circles, leg swings).

- **HIIT Circuit:**

    - 20 seconds of high knees

    - 20 seconds of squat jumps

    - 20 seconds of push-ups

    - 20 seconds of bicycle crunches

- **Rest:** 10 seconds

- Repeat the circuit 5 times.

- **Cool down:** 5 minutes of static stretching.

Tabata Protocol Workout:

- **Warm up:** 5 minutes of light jogging or cycling.

- **Tabata Intervals:**

    - 20 seconds of jump squats

    - 10 seconds of rest

    - 20 seconds of push-ups

    - 10 seconds of rest

    - Repeat for 4 minutes (8 rounds total).

- **Cool down:** 5 minutes of stretching.

Cardio HIIT Workout:

- **Warm up:** 5 minutes of brisk walking or jogging.

- **HIIT Circuit:**
    - 30 seconds of sprinting
    - 30 seconds of walking or jogging
    - Repeat for 10-15 minutes.
- **Cool down:** 5 minutes of walking and stretching.

Dumbbell HIIT Workout:

- **Warm up:** 5 minutes of dynamic movements (e.g., arm circles, leg swings).
- **HIIT Circuit:**
    - 20 seconds of dumbbell thrusters
    - 20 seconds of dumbbell rows
    - 20 seconds of dumbbell lunges
    - 20 seconds of dumbbell shoulder presses
- **Rest:** 10 seconds
- Repeat the circuit 5 times.
- **Cool down:** 5 minutes of static stretching.

Plyometric HIIT Workout:

- **Warm up:** 5 minutes of light cardio (e.g., jumping jacks, high knees).
- **HIIT Circuit:**
    - 30 seconds of box jumps
    - 30 seconds of plyometric push-ups

- 30 seconds of jumping lunges
  - 30 seconds of burpee broad jumps
- **Rest:** 30 seconds
- Repeat the circuit 3-4 times.
- **Cool down:** 5 minutes of stretching.

These are just a few examples of HIIT workouts that you can incorporate into your fitness routine. Feel free to modify the exercises, duration, and intensity based on your fitness level and preferences. Always listen to your body and consult with a healthcare professional before starting any new exercise program, especially if you have any underlying health conditions.

Chapter 14: Understanding Anatomy: Your Body's Blueprint

In the heart of the bustling city, Emily sat at her desk, frustrated and discouraged. Despite her dedication to exercise and healthy eating, she struggled to see the results she desired. Feeling defeated, she confided in her friend, Jennifer, a personal trainer with a passion for anatomy.

"Emily," Jennifer said gently, "have you ever considered the importance of understanding your body's anatomy in achieving your fitness goals?"

Perplexed, Emily listened as Jennifer explained the intricate relationship between muscles, bones, and movement. Jennifer emphasized that knowledge of anatomy could significantly impact the effectiveness of workouts and lead to better results.

Intrigued, Emily decided to delve deeper into the world of anatomy. She spent hours studying muscle groups, joint mechanics, and movement patterns, eager to apply her newfound knowledge to her fitness journey.

Armed with a deeper understanding of anatomy, Emily adjusted her workout routine to target specific muscle groups more effectively. She incorporated compound exercises like squats, deadlifts, and push-ups to engage multiple muscles simultaneously, maximizing her calorie burn and muscle activation.

As Emily's workouts became more targeted and efficient, she began to see noticeable improvements in her strength, endurance, and physique. With each workout, she felt more connected to her body, understanding how each movement contributed to her overall fitness goals.

Not only did understanding anatomy enhance Emily's workouts, but it also helped her prevent injuries and overcome plateaus. By identifying muscular imbalances and movement dysfunctions, she was able to correct them through targeted exercises and proper form, allowing her to progress more effectively towards her goals.

With newfound confidence and a deeper appreciation for her body's capabilities, Emily continued on her fitness journey with renewed vigor. She no longer viewed exercise as a chore but rather as a celebration of her body's incredible potential.

Through the power of understanding anatomy, Emily unlocked new levels of success in her fitness journey, proving that knowledge truly is power when it comes to achieving our weight loss and fitness goals.

Understanding anatomical differences between men and women can help tailor exercise routines and weight loss strategies for optimal results. Here are some key examples:

Muscle Composition:

- Men generally have a higher percentage of muscle mass compared to women due to differences in hormonal profiles, particularly higher levels of testosterone.
- Women tend to have a higher percentage of type I muscle fibers, which are more resistant to fatigue and better suited for endurance activities.
- Tailoring workouts to capitalize on these differences can help men focus on strength and power training, while women may benefit from incorporating more endurance-based exercises.

Body Fat Distribution:

- Men typically store fat in the abdominal region (android or "apple-shaped" distribution), while women tend to store fat in the hips, thighs, and buttocks (gynoid or "pear-shaped" distribution).
- Targeted exercises that address these specific areas can help individuals achieve their desired body composition goals. For example, men may focus on core and abdominal exercises, while women may incorporate exercises to target the lower body.

Pelvic Structure:

- Women have wider pelvic bones and a greater angle of the pelvis compared to men, which can influence lower body mechanics and alignment during exercises such as squats and lunges.
- It's important for both men and women to maintain proper form and alignment during lower body exercises to prevent injury and maximize effectiveness.

Hormonal Influences:

- Hormonal fluctuations throughout the menstrual cycle can affect energy levels, muscle recovery, and metabolism in women. Understanding these fluctuations can help women optimize their workout schedule and nutrition to align with their hormonal phases.
- Menopause-related hormonal changes in women can also impact metabolism and body composition, requiring adjustments in exercise and dietary habits to support weight loss and muscle maintenance.

Nutritional Needs:

- Men typically have higher calorie and protein requirements due to greater muscle mass and metabolic rates. Adequate protein intake is essential for muscle repair and growth in both men and women, but the specific amounts may vary.

- Women may have increased iron requirements due to menstrual blood loss, while men may need to monitor zinc and magnesium intake for optimal testosterone production.

By understanding these anatomical differences, individuals can tailor their exercise routines, nutritional strategies, and weight loss approaches to better suit their unique physiological needs and goals. Consulting with a qualified fitness professional or healthcare provider can provide further guidance on optimizing exercise and nutrition for men and women.

Chapter 15: Nutrition Essentials: Fueling Your Transformation

Nestled among the hustle and bustle of city life, lived two neighbors: Erika and Mike. While outwardly they appeared similar, their daily routines and eating habits couldn't be more different.

Erika, a busy marketing executive, often found herself skipping meals or reaching for convenient but unhealthy snacks throughout the day. Her diet consisted mainly of processed foods, fast food takeout, and sugary treats grabbed on the go. Despite her demanding schedule, Erika struggled with low energy levels, frequent mood swings, and digestive issues.

On the other hand, Mike, a software engineer with a passion for health and fitness, approached nutrition with mindfulness and intention. He prioritized whole, nutrient-dense foods, including lean proteins, colorful fruits and vegetables, whole grains, and healthy fats. Mike took the time to plan and prepare balanced meals, even amid his busy work schedule.

As weeks turned into months, the stark contrast in their nutritional choices became increasingly evident. While Erika continued to battle fatigue, mood fluctuations, and digestive discomfort, Mike thrived with sustained energy, mental clarity, and a positive outlook on life.

One sunny afternoon, Erika confided in Mike about her struggles with energy levels and overall well-being. Mike listened attentively, empathizing with her challenges, and gently shared his own experiences with prioritizing nutrition.

Inspired by Mike's example, Erika decided to embark on a journey of nutritional transformation. She began incorporating more whole foods into her diet, gradually replacing processed snacks with nourishing alternatives. With each meal, she focused on balance and variety, savoring the flavors and textures of fresh, wholesome ingredients.

As the days passed, Erika noticed subtle but significant changes in how she felt. Her energy levels stabilized, her mood improved, and her digestive issues gradually resolved. She found herself more focused and productive at work, with a newfound sense of vitality and well-being.

With each passing day, Erika became more attuned to the profound impact that proper nutrition could have on her daily life. She marveled at the power of food to nourish not only her body but also her mind and spirit. Through mindful eating and a commitment to nourishing herself from the inside out, Erika discovered a newfound sense of vitality, joy, and fulfillment in her daily life.

As the sun set on their neighborhood that evening, Erika and Mike shared a moment of gratitude for the transformative power of proper nutrition. Their journey had not only enriched their own lives but also inspired those around them to embrace the profound impact of healthy eating on their daily well-being and quality of life.

Why is Understanding Proper Nutrition So Important?
Proper nutrition plays a crucial role in fueling our bodies to feel and perform better, both physically and mentally. Here's a scientific breakdown of how this process works:

Energy Production:
- Carbohydrates are the body's primary source of energy. They are broken down into glucose, which is then transported to cells throughout the body to fuel various functions.
- Additionally, fats provide a concentrated source of energy, especially during prolonged or low-intensity activities. They are broken down into fatty acids, which are converted into energy through a process called beta-oxidation.

Muscle Repair and Growth:

- Protein is essential for repairing and building muscle tissue. During exercise, muscle fibers undergo microscopic damage, and consuming adequate protein post-workout helps to repair and rebuild these fibers, leading to muscle growth and strength gains.
- Amino acids, the building blocks of protein, play a critical role in this process. Consuming a variety of protein sources ensures a sufficient intake of all essential amino acids necessary for muscle repair and growth.

Nutrient Delivery:

- Vitamins and minerals serve as cofactors in numerous metabolic processes, including energy production, muscle contraction, and immune function. Consuming a diverse range of fruits, vegetables, whole grains, and lean proteins ensures an adequate intake of these micronutrients, facilitating optimal nutrient delivery throughout the body.

Hydration and Fluid Balance:

- Water is essential for maintaining proper hydration and fluid balance in the body. During exercise, the body loses fluids through sweat, and adequate hydration is crucial for regulating body temperature, lubricating joints, and transporting nutrients and oxygen to cells.
- Electrolytes such as sodium, potassium, and chloride are also lost through sweat and need to be replenished to maintain proper fluid balance and electrolyte levels.

Brain Function and Mental Well-being:

- Nutrients such as omega-3 fatty acids, vitamins B6, B12, and folate, and minerals like iron and zinc play key roles in supporting brain function and mental well-being.
- Omega-3 fatty acids, found in fatty fish, flaxseeds, and walnuts, are particularly important for cognitive function, mood regulation, and reducing inflammation in the brain.

Immune Function:

- Proper nutrition supports a healthy immune system by providing essential nutrients needed for immune cell production and function. Key nutrients include vitamins A, C, D, E, zinc, and selenium, which help to strengthen the immune response and protect against infections and illnesses.

In summary, proper nutrition provides the essential nutrients needed to fuel our bodies, support physical performance, promote muscle repair and growth, maintain hydration and fluid balance, support brain function and mental well-being, and strengthen immune function. By nourishing our bodies with a balanced and varied diet, we can optimize our health, energy levels, and overall well-being.

Chapter 16: Ancient Wisdom, Modern Results: Timeless Remedies

In the heart of a remote village nestled among rolling hills, lived an elderly woman named Ana. Widely revered for her wisdom and healing prowess, Ana was known throughout the village as the guardian of ancient health remedies passed down through generations.

As the sun dipped below the horizon, casting a warm glow over the village, young Mia sought out Ana's humble abode. Mia, weary from the weight of her struggles with weight loss and fitness, hoped to find solace and guidance in Ana's ancient wisdom.

With a gentle smile, Ana welcomed Mia into her home, her eyes twinkling with knowledge and kindness. Sensing Mia's longing for answers, Ana beckoned her to sit by the crackling fire, where stories of healing and transformation unfolded.

"Long ago," Ana began, her voice a soothing melody, "our ancestors understood the profound connection between nature, nourishment, and vitality. They harnessed the power of herbs, spices, and rituals to heal the body, mind, and spirit."

With a twinkle in her eye, Ana shared tales of ancient remedies passed down through the ages. She spoke of the healing properties of turmeric, ginger, and cinnamon, revered for their ability to support metabolism, digestion, and weight management.

Ana recounted stories of herbal teas brewed from fragrant leaves and flowers, their soothing aromas infusing the air with tranquility and healing energy. She spoke of rituals practiced under the light of the full moon, invoking ancient wisdom to cleanse the body of toxins and stagnant energy.

As Mia listened, she felt a sense of wonder and hope stirring within her soul. Could these ancient remedies hold the key to unlocking her own journey of healing and transformation?

Inspired by Ana's wisdom, Mia embarked on a journey of exploration and discovery, eager to embrace the ancient remedies that had stood the test of time. She sought out fragrant herbs and spices, brewing nourishing potions and elixirs to support her body's natural balance and vitality.

With each sip of herbal tea, Mia felt a renewed sense of energy and clarity coursing through her veins. She embraced rituals of self-care and mindfulness, honoring her body as a sacred vessel of health and well-being.

As the seasons turned and the earth blossomed with new life, Mia's journey of healing and transformation blossomed alongside it. With each passing day, she felt lighter, stronger, and more radiant than ever before.

In the ancient wisdom of Ana and the healing power of nature, Mia found the keys to unlocking her own path to weight loss and fitness. With gratitude in her heart and a newfound sense of empowerment, she embraced the ancient remedies that had guided her on this transformative journey, knowing that the wisdom of the ages would forever illuminate her path forward.

Ancient Remedies for Modern-Day Ailments

Here's a list of ancient herbal remedies that have been traditionally used to help with weight loss and promote longevity, along with brief explanations of their benefits:

Turmeric:

- Turmeric contains curcumin, a compound with powerful anti-inflammatory and antioxidant properties. It may support weight loss by reducing inflammation, improving insulin sensitivity, and boosting metabolism.

Ginger:

- Ginger is known for its ability to aid digestion, reduce appetite, and increase thermogenesis (the body's ability to burn calories). It may also help regulate blood sugar levels and reduce inflammation, supporting overall health and weight management.

Cinnamon:

- Cinnamon has been shown to help regulate blood sugar levels by improving insulin sensitivity and reducing insulin resistance. It may also enhance metabolism and promote fat loss, making it a valuable addition to weight loss diets.

Green Tea:

- Green tea is rich in catechins, antioxidants that have been found to increase metabolism and promote fat oxidation. It may also help suppress appetite and reduce the absorption of fat, leading to greater weight loss and improved health.

Ginseng:

- Ginseng has adaptogenic properties, meaning it helps the body adapt to stress and maintain balance. It may support weight loss by reducing stress-related cravings, increasing energy levels, and improving overall vitality and well-being.

Fenugreek:

- Fenugreek seeds are rich in soluble fiber, which can help promote feelings of fullness and reduce appetite. They may also help regulate blood sugar levels and improve insulin sensitivity, supporting weight loss and metabolic health.

Garcinia Cambogia:

- Garcinia cambogia contains hydroxycitric acid (HCA), which has been shown to inhibit the enzyme responsible for converting carbohydrates into fat. It may also help suppress appetite and increase fat metabolism, making it a popular ingredient in weight loss supplements.

Holy Basil (Tulsi):

- Holy basil is revered for its adaptogenic and stress-relieving properties. It may help reduce stress-related eating, balance cortisol levels, and support overall health and longevity.

Dandelion:

- Dandelion has diuretic properties, meaning it helps the body eliminate excess water and reduce bloating. It may also support liver health and digestion, making it a valuable herb for weight loss and detoxification.

Licorice Root:

- Licorice root contains compounds that may help regulate cortisol levels and reduce stress-related cravings. It may also support adrenal health and improve energy levels, promoting overall vitality and well-being.

These ancient herbal remedies have been valued for centuries for their potent medicinal properties and ability to support weight loss, metabolism, and overall longevity. Incorporating them into a balanced diet and healthy lifestyle may offer numerous health benefits and contribute to a longer, healthier life.

It's important to consider other factors like herbs as part of maintaining a healthy lifestyle because they offer a holistic approach to health and wellness. While factors like diet and exercise are crucial, integrating herbal remedies can provide additional support and balance to the body, mind, and spirit. Here's why it's essential to consider herbs:

1. **Comprehensive Health Support:** Herbs contain a variety of bioactive compounds that can offer a wide range of health benefits beyond basic nutrition. They may possess antioxidant, anti-inflammatory, antimicrobial, and adaptogenic properties, which can support various aspects of health, including immune function, stress management, and detoxification.

2. **Traditional Wisdom:** Herbal remedies have been used for centuries in traditional medicine systems around the world, including Ayurveda, Traditional Chinese Medicine (TCM), and Indigenous healing practices. Drawing upon this ancient wisdom allows us to tap into centuries of accumulated knowledge about the healing properties of plants and their synergistic effects on the body.

3. **Individualized Approach:** Herbs offer a personalized approach to health and wellness, allowing individuals to tailor their herbal regimen to their unique needs, preferences, and health goals. Whether addressing specific health concerns or promoting overall well-being, herbs can be customized to support individual biochemistry and constitution.

4. **Natural and Sustainable:** Herbs are derived from natural sources, making them a safe and sustainable option for health promotion and disease prevention. Unlike synthetic pharmaceuticals, which may come with unwanted side effects and environmental concerns, herbs offer a gentle and environmentally friendly approach to health care.

5. **Enhanced Nutrient Absorption**: Certain herbs can enhance nutrient absorption and utilization, making them valuable additions to a healthy diet. For example, herbs like black pepper may improve the bioavailability of nutrients like curcumin in turmeric, maximizing their therapeutic effects on the body.

6. **Mind-Body Connection**: Many herbs have a profound impact on mental and emotional well-being, helping to calm the mind, reduce stress, and promote relaxation. By addressing the mind-body connection, herbs can support holistic health and create a sense of balance and harmony within the body.

Overall, integrating herbs into a healthy lifestyle can provide a multifaceted approach to health promotion, addressing not only physical health but also mental, emotional, and spiritual well-being. By harnessing the power of nature's pharmacy, individuals can optimize their health and vitality, leading to a more vibrant and fulfilling life.

Chapter 17: Meal Prep Mastery: Planning for Success

Amid the daily grind of work and responsibilities, lived two individuals: Mark and Emily. Both had struggled with their weight for years, feeling trapped in cycles of fad diets and unhealthy eating habits. However, their lives took a transformative turn when they discovered the power of meal prep to take control of their portions and nourish their bodies with healthy, nutritious food.

Mark, a busy executive, often found himself reaching for convenience foods and takeout meals during hectic workdays. Despite his efforts to eat healthier, he struggled to control his portions and make balanced choices. Frustrated by his lack of progress, Mark decided to try meal prepping as a solution.

Emily, a dedicated nurse, faced similar challenges with her weight and nutrition. Long shifts at the hospital left her little time or energy to cook healthy meals, leading to frequent indulgence in fast food and processed snacks. Determined to take charge of her health, Emily turned to meal prep as a way to prioritize nutritious eating amidst her demanding schedule.

Armed with determination and a newfound commitment to health, Mark and Emily embarked on their meal prep journeys. They set aside time each week to plan and prepare their meals in advance, focusing on balanced combinations of lean proteins, whole grains, and colorful fruits and vegetables.

As the weeks passed, Mark and Emily began to experience remarkable transformations in their bodies and minds. By controlling their portions and eating balanced meals, they felt more satisfied and energized throughout the day. They no longer succumbed to cravings for unhealthy snacks or overeating at mealtimes.

With each passing week, Mark and Emily stepped on the scale with anticipation, eager to see the results of their efforts. To their amazement, the numbers on the scale began to drop steadily, reflecting the pounds they had shed through mindful eating and portion control.

After three months of consistent meal prep, Mark had lost 20 pounds, while Emily had lost 15 pounds. Not only had they achieved their weight loss goals, but they also felt healthier, happier, and more confident than ever before.

Their success inspired those around them to adopt healthier eating habits and prioritize meal prep as a tool for weight loss and overall well-being. Together, Mark and Emily proved that with dedication, planning, and a commitment to nourishing their bodies with wholesome food, anything was possible.

Through the simple act of meal prep, Mark and Emily had unlocked the secret to sustainable weight loss and a lifetime of health and vitality. With each nutritious meal they prepared, they took another step forward on their journey to a healthier, happier life.Here's a guide to proper meal prep and daily nutritional needs:

Meal Prep Guidelines:

1. **Plan Your Meals:** Take some time each week to plan your meals in advance. Consider your schedule, nutritional needs, and personal preferences when choosing recipes.

2. **Choose Nutrient-Dense Foods:** Focus on incorporating a variety of nutrient-dense foods into your meals, including lean proteins, whole grains, fruits, vegetables, and healthy fats.

3. **Portion Control:** Use portion control to ensure balanced meals and prevent overeating. Invest in portion-controlled containers or use a food scale to measure serving sizes accurately.

4. **Cook in Bulk:** Cook large batches of staple foods such as grains, proteins, and vegetables to use as building blocks for your meals throughout the week. This can save time and make meal prep more efficient.

5. **Include Variety:** Aim for variety in your meals to ensure you get a wide range of nutrients. Experiment with different flavors, textures, and cuisines to keep meals exciting and enjoyable.

6. **Packaging and Storage**: Store prepared meals in airtight containers in the refrigerator or freezer to maintain freshness and prevent spoilage. Label containers with the date and contents for easy identification.

Daily Nutritional Needs:

1. **Macronutrients:**

- **Protein:** Aim to consume a sufficient amount of protein to support muscle repair and growth. The recommended daily intake is around 0.8 grams of protein per kilogram of body weight for sedentary individuals, and higher for those who are physically active or trying to build muscle.

- **Carbohydrates:** Choose complex carbohydrates such as whole grains, fruits, and vegetables for sustained energy and fiber intake. The recommended daily intake varies depending on individual factors such as activity level and metabolism.

- **Fats:** Include sources of healthy fats such as avocados, nuts, seeds, and olive oil in your diet for heart health and satiety. Aim to limit saturated and trans fats found in processed and fried foods.

2. **Micronutrients:**

- **Vitamins**: Consume a variety of fruits, vegetables, and whole grains to ensure an adequate intake of vitamins, including vitamin A, vitamin C, vitamin D, and B vitamins.

- **Minerals**: Include sources of minerals such as calcium, magnesium, potassium, and iron in your diet through foods like dairy products, leafy greens, nuts, seeds, and lean meats.

3. **Hydration:** Drink plenty of water throughout the day to stay hydrated and support optimal bodily functions. Aim for at least 8 glasses (64 ounces) of water per day, or more if you are physically active or in a hot climate.

4. **Fiber:** Incorporate sources of dietary fiber such as fruits, vegetables, whole grains, legumes, and nuts into your meals to support digestive health and promote feelings of fullness.

5. **Antioxidants:** Include foods rich in antioxidants such as berries, leafy greens, nuts, seeds, and colorful vegetables to protect against oxidative stress and inflammation.

By following these meal prep guidelines and meeting your daily nutritional needs, you can support your overall health, energy levels, and well-being. Remember to listen to your body's hunger and fullness cues, and make adjustments to your meal plan as needed to ensure it meets your individual needs and preferences.

Here are some examples of healthy meals you can prep:

Breakfast:

1. **Overnight oats**: Combine rolled oats with milk (or a plant-based alternative), Greek yogurt, chia seeds, and a dash of honey or maple syrup. Add toppings such as sliced fruit, nuts, and seeds. Portion into jars and refrigerate overnight for a quick and nutritious breakfast.

2. **Egg muffins:** Whisk together eggs, chopped vegetables (such as bell peppers, spinach, and tomatoes), and cheese. Pour the mixture into muffin tins and bake until set. Store in the refrigerator and reheat in the morning for a protein-packed breakfast on the go.

Lunch:

1. **Grilled chicken salad:** Grill chicken breasts and slice thinly. Prepare a bed of mixed greens and top with sliced chicken, cherry tomatoes, cucumber slices, avocado, and a drizzle of balsamic vinaigrette. Portion into containers for a fresh and satisfying lunch option.

2. **Quinoa and vegetable stir-fry**: Cook quinoa according to package instructions. In a skillet, sauté chopped vegetables (such as broccoli, bell peppers, carrots, and snap peas) with

garlic and ginger. Add cooked quinoa and a splash of soy sauce or teriyaki sauce. Divide into containers for a colorful and nutritious meal.

Dinner:

1. **Baked salmon with roasted vegetables**: Season salmon fillets with olive oil, lemon juice, and herbs (such as dill or parsley). Place on a baking sheet alongside chopped vegetables (such as asparagus, zucchini, and cherry tomatoes). Roast in the oven until salmon is cooked through and vegetables are tender. Serve with a side of quinoa or brown rice.

2. **Turkey and black bean chili:** Brown ground turkey in a large pot with onions, garlic, and chili powder. Add canned black beans, diced tomatoes, low-sodium chicken broth, and your favorite chili spices. Simmer until flavors meld together. Portion into containers and garnish with Greek yogurt, avocado slices, and cilantro.

Snacks:

1. **Greek yogurt with berries and almonds**: Portion Greek yogurt into small containers and top with fresh berries and a sprinkle of almonds. This snack provides a balance of protein, fiber, and healthy fats to keep you satisfied between meals.

2. **Hummus and vegetable sticks:** Portion hummus into small containers and pack with carrot sticks, cucumber slices, bell pepper strips, and cherry tomatoes. This crunchy and satisfying snack is perfect for dipping and provides a dose of vitamins and minerals.

These are just a few examples of healthy meals you can prep ahead of time to support your nutrition goals and save time during busy weekdays. Feel free to customize the recipes based on your dietary preferences and ingredient availability!

Chapter 18: Yoga for Weight Loss: Finding Balance

Tiffany was caught in the cyclical chaos of daily life, living as a young professional trapped in a whirlwind of deadlines, stress, and unhealthy habits. Day after day, she found herself trapped in a cycle of sedentary work, fast food lunches, and restless nights filled with anxiety and tension.

Feeling the weight of her hectic lifestyle bearing down on her, Tiffany knew she needed to make a change. Seeking solace and a sense of balance, she stumbled upon a yoga studio nestled in a quiet corner of the city. Intrigued by the promise of inner peace and physical rejuvenation, Tiffany tentatively stepped inside, uncertain of what lay ahead.

As she unrolled her mat and settled into her first downward dog, Tiffany felt a wave of apprehension wash over her. The unfamiliar poses and rhythmic flow of breath seemed daunting at first, but she pushed through her doubts, guided by the soothing voice of the instructor and the gentle encouragement of her fellow yogis.

With each practice, Tiffany felt herself growing stronger, both physically and mentally. The slow, deliberate movements of yoga helped her release tension stored in her body, easing the knots of stress that had accumulated over years of neglect. As she delved deeper into her practice, Tiffany discovered newfound strength and flexibility she never knew she possessed.

But the benefits of yoga extended far beyond the physical realm. With each mindful breath and meditative moment, Tiffany found herself reconnecting with her inner self, tapping into a wellspring of calm and clarity that had long eluded her. The practice of yoga became her sanctuary, a sacred space where she could quiet the noise of the outside world and listen to the whispers of her own heart.

As weeks turned into months, Tiffany's dedication to her yoga practice began to yield remarkable results. Her body grew leaner and more toned, shedding the weight of stress and unhealthy habits that had held her back for so long. She found herself making healthier choices, nourishing her body with wholesome foods and prioritizing self-care in ways she never thought possible.

But perhaps the greatest transformation of all was the newfound sense of empowerment and self-love that blossomed within her. Through yoga, Tiffany learned to embrace her body as a vessel of strength and resilience, worthy of love and respect. She let go of the need for perfection, embracing the beauty of imperfection and finding joy in the journey of self-discovery.

With each step on her yoga mat, Tiffany forged a path towards a healthier, happier life, one breath at a time. In the sanctuary of the yoga studio, she found not only physical strength and flexibility but also a sense of peace and purpose that illuminated her path forward. And as she flowed through her practice with grace and gratitude, Tiffany knew that she had found her home in the practice of yoga—a journey of transformation that would continue to unfold, one pose at a time.

Different Styles of Yoga

For beginners, it's important to choose yoga styles that are accessible, gentle, and beginner-friendly. Here are some of the best types of yoga for beginners:

1. **Hatha Yoga:** Hatha yoga is a gentle and slow-paced practice that focuses on basic yoga poses and breathing techniques. It's great for beginners as it provides a solid foundation and helps build strength, flexibility, and mindfulness.

2. **Vinyasa Yoga:** Vinyasa yoga, also known as flow yoga, involves linking breath with movement in a dynamic and flowing sequence of poses. While it can be challenging, many vinyasa classes offer modifications and options for beginners, making it suitable for those who are new to yoga.

3. **Yin Yoga:** Yin yoga is a slow and meditative practice that involves holding passive stretches for extended periods,

typically ranging from 1 to 5 minutes. It targets the connective tissues of the body, promoting flexibility, relaxation, and deep release. Yin yoga is excellent for beginners as it allows for gentle exploration of the body's limitations and encourages introspection and mindfulness.

4. **Iyengar Yoga:** Iyengar yoga focuses on precise alignment and uses props such as blocks, straps, and blankets to support the body in various poses. This style of yoga is excellent for beginners as it helps build strength, flexibility, and body awareness while reducing the risk of injury.

5. **Restorative Yoga:** Restorative yoga is a deeply relaxing practice that involves holding supported poses for extended periods, allowing the body to completely relax and release tension. It's ideal for beginners who may be dealing with stress, fatigue, or chronic pain, as it promotes deep relaxation and rejuvenation.

6. **Kundalini Yoga:** Kundalini yoga combines dynamic movements, breathwork, chanting, and meditation to awaken energy and promote spiritual growth. While it may seem intimidating at first, many Kundalini classes offer accessible options for beginners, making it suitable for

those who are new to yoga and seeking a holistic approach to well-being.

Remember to listen to your body and honor your limitations as you explore different styles of yoga. It's essential to find a practice that resonates with you and supports your physical, mental, and emotional needs as a beginner yogi.

Best Yoga Poses for Begginers:

1. **Mountain Pose (Tadasana):** Stand tall with feet hip-width apart, arms by your sides, and palms facing forward. Root down through your feet, lengthen your spine, and lift through the crown of your head. Engage your core and breathe deeply.

2. **Downward-Facing Dog (Adho Mukha Svanasana):** Start on your hands and knees, then lift your hips up and back, straightening your arms and legs to form an inverted V shape. Press your palms into the mat, engage your core, and lengthen through your spine. Keep your heels reaching toward the ground.

3. **Child's Pose (Balasana):** Kneel on the mat with your big toes touching and knees hip-width apart. Lower your torso

between your thighs and extend your arms forward, resting your forehead on the mat. Relax your shoulders, breathe deeply, and allow your body to release tension.

4. **Warrior I (Virabhadrasana I)**: Step one foot back into a lunge position, with your front knee bent at a 90-degree angle and your back leg straight. Square your hips forward and raise your arms overhead, reaching toward the sky. Keep your chest lifted and gaze forward.

5. **Warrior II (Virabhadrasana II)**: From Warrior I, open your hips and arms out to the sides, parallel to the mat. Keep your front knee bent and aligned with your ankle, and gaze over your front fingertips. Engage your core and sink deeper into the lunge.

6. **Tree Pose (Vrksasana):** Stand tall with feet hip-width apart and arms by your sides. Shift your weight onto one foot and place the sole of your other foot on the inner thigh or calf of your standing leg. Bring your palms together at your heart center or extend them overhead. Find a focal point to help with balance and breathe deeply.

7. **Seated Forward Fold (Paschimottanasana)**: Sit on the mat with your legs extended in front of you and feet flexed. Inhale to lengthen your spine, then exhale to hinge at the

hips and fold forward, reaching for your feet or shins. Keep your back straight and gaze forward, relaxing into the stretch.

8. **Bridge Pose (Setu Bandhasana):** Lie on your back with knees bent and feet hip-width apart, arms by your sides. Press into your feet and lift your hips toward the ceiling, engaging your glutes and core. Keep your shoulders grounded and interlace your fingers beneath your back for support.

9. **Corpse Pose (Savasana):** Lie on your back with legs extended and arms by your sides, palms facing up. Close your eyes and relax your entire body, allowing yourself to surrender to the ground. Focus on your breath and let go of any tension or stress.

These beginner-friendly yoga poses are accessible and offer a range of benefits, including improved flexibility, strength, balance, and relaxation. Remember to listen to your body and modify as needed to ensure a safe and enjoyable practice.

Health Benefits of Group Yoga Lessons

Joining group yoga lessons regularly can offer numerous benefits for creating a healthier lifestyle. Here are some of the key advantages:

1. **Community Support:** Practicing yoga in a group setting provides a sense of community and support. You'll have the opportunity to connect with like-minded individuals who share similar health and wellness goals, fostering a sense of belonging and camaraderie.

2. **Motivation and Accountability:** Attending regular group yoga classes can help keep you motivated and accountable to your practice. Knowing that you have a class scheduled and friends to practice with can encourage you to prioritize your health and make consistent efforts toward your wellness goals.

3. **Structured Routine:** Group yoga classes offer a structured routine and dedicated time for self-care. By committing to regular class attendance, you can establish a healthy habit and incorporate yoga into your weekly schedule, promoting consistency and progress in your practice.

4. **Professional Guidance:** In a group yoga setting, you'll receive guidance and instruction from experienced yoga

teachers who can offer personalized feedback and adjustments to support your practice. Their expertise can help you refine your alignment, deepen your poses, and avoid injury as you progress on your yoga journey.

5. **Variety and Exploration:** Group yoga classes often offer a variety of styles, levels, and class formats to choose from, allowing you to explore different aspects of yoga and find what resonates with you. Whether you prefer a gentle flow, a challenging vinyasa class, or a restorative practice, there's something for everyone in a group setting.

6. **Physical Benefits:** Regular participation in group yoga classes can lead to a wide range of physical benefits, including improved flexibility, strength, balance, and posture. Yoga poses and sequences work to stretch and strengthen the muscles, lubricate the joints, and increase overall mobility and range of motion.

7. **Stress Reduction**: Yoga is known for its stress-relieving effects on the body and mind. Group classes provide a supportive environment for relaxation and mindfulness, allowing you to release tension, quiet the mind, and cultivate a sense of inner peace and calm amidst life's challenges.

8. **Emotional Well-being:** In addition to its physical benefits, yoga can also promote emotional well-being and mental clarity. Group classes offer opportunities for self-reflection, self-expression, and emotional release, helping you to cultivate greater self-awareness, resilience, and emotional balance.

Overall, joining group yoga lessons regularly can be a powerful catalyst for creating a healthier lifestyle, supporting your physical, mental, and emotional well-being, and fostering a sense of connection and community along the way.

Chapter 19: Sleep and Weight: Restoring Harmony

In a bustling city where the lights never dim and the streets never sleep, lived a young woman named Emma. Like many urban dwellers, Emma led a fast-paced life filled with work deadlines, social engagements, and endless distractions. Despite her hectic schedule, Emma cherished her nightly routine—a fleeting moment of peace amidst the chaos.

However, despite her best efforts, Emma struggled to achieve restful sleep night after night. Tossing and turning, she found herself trapped in a cycle of insomnia and exhaustion, unable to escape the grasp of sleeplessness. Little did she know, her restless nights were taking a toll on more than just her energy levels—they were also wreaking havoc on her weight and overall health.

As weeks turned into months, Emma began to notice subtle changes in her body and mood. Despite her healthy eating habits and regular exercise routine, she found herself gaining weight inexplicably, her clothes fitting tighter and her energy levels plummeting. Frustrated and perplexed, Emma turned to her doctor for answers.

After a series of tests and examinations, Emma's doctor revealed a startling truth—her chronic sleep deprivation was at the root of her health woes. It wasn't just a matter of feeling tired and groggy—it was a matter of hormonal imbalance, metabolic disruption, and increased risk of chronic disease.

Emma learned that poor sleep can disrupt the delicate balance of hormones that regulate appetite and metabolism, leading to increased cravings for sugary, high-calorie foods and decreased feelings of fullness. As a result, she found herself reaching for unhealthy snacks late at night, seeking comfort in food to cope with her sleepless nights.

Furthermore, inadequate sleep wreaked havoc on Emma's body's ability to regulate blood sugar levels, increasing her risk of insulin resistance and type 2 diabetes. It also disrupted her body's natural circadian rhythms, leading to imbalances in hormones such as cortisol and leptin, which play a crucial role in regulating metabolism and appetite.

But perhaps the most alarming revelation was the link between chronic sleep deprivation and weight gain. Studies have shown that individuals who consistently get less sleep are more likely to be overweight or obese compared to those who get adequate rest. This is due in part to the disruption of appetite-regulating hormones and metabolic processes, as well as the negative impact on energy expenditure and physical activity levels.

Armed with this newfound knowledge, Emma embarked on a mission to prioritize her sleep and reclaim her health. She implemented a bedtime routine that included relaxation techniques such as meditation and deep breathing, created a sleep-friendly environment free of distractions and electronic devices, and established a consistent sleep schedule.

Slowly but surely, Emma began to notice improvements in her sleep quality and overall well-being. Her energy levels soared, her mood stabilized, and, most importantly, her weight began to normalize. By prioritizing her sleep and addressing the root cause of her health issues, Emma was able to reclaim control of her life and pave the way for a healthier, happier future.

As Emma drifted off to sleep each night, she reflected on the profound impact that restful slumber had on her weight and overall health. No longer did she view sleep as a luxury—it was a necessity, a vital component of her journey toward optimal well-being. And as she closed her eyes and surrendered to the embrace of sleep, Emma knew that she was taking an important step toward a healthier, happier life.

Understanding the Impratnace of Proper Sleep and Weight Management

Regular, restful sleep plays a critical role in maintaining overall health and managing weight effectively. Here are some scientific health benefits of regular sleep and its impact on weight management, along with advice for improving sleep quality:

Health Benefits of Regular Sleep:

1. **Hormonal Regulation:** Adequate sleep helps regulate hormones that control appetite and metabolism, such as leptin and ghrelin. Leptin signals fullness to the brain, while ghrelin stimulates hunger. Poor sleep disrupts the balance of these hormones, leading to increased appetite and cravings for high-calorie foods.

2. **Metabolic Function:** Sleep deprivation can impair glucose metabolism and insulin sensitivity, increasing the risk of weight gain and type 2 diabetes. Getting enough sleep supports optimal metabolic function, aiding in the regulation of blood sugar levels and energy balance.

3. **Energy Levels:** Quality sleep is essential for replenishing energy stores and supporting physical and cognitive performance. Adequate rest allows the body to repair and regenerate tissues, promoting vitality and productivity throughout the day.

4. **Stress Reduction:** Sleep plays a crucial role in managing stress levels and promoting emotional well-being. Chronic

sleep deprivation can increase levels of stress hormones like cortisol, which may contribute to weight gain and metabolic dysfunction over time.

5. **Appetite Regulation:** Sleep influences the brain's reward system and decision-making processes, affecting food choices and eating behaviors. Lack of sleep can lead to impulsive food cravings and overeating, making it more challenging to maintain a healthy diet and weight.

Advice for Improving Sleep Quality:

1. **Establish a Bedtime Routine**: Create a consistent bedtime routine to signal to your body that it's time to wind down and prepare for sleep. Engage in relaxing activities such as reading, gentle stretching, or meditation to promote relaxation and reduce stress.

2. **Create a Sleep-Friendly Environment:** Make your bedroom conducive to sleep by keeping it dark, quiet, and cool. Invest in a comfortable mattress and pillows, and remove electronic devices that emit blue light, which can disrupt the production of sleep hormones.

3. **Limit Caffeine and Alcohol:** Avoid consuming caffeine and alcohol close to bedtime, as they can interfere with

sleep quality and disrupt your natural sleep-wake cycle. Opt for caffeine-free herbal teas or warm milk instead.

4. **Practice Stress Management:** Incorporate stress-reducing techniques into your daily routine, such as deep breathing exercises, progressive muscle relaxation, or mindfulness meditation. Managing stress can improve sleep quality and support overall health and well-being.

5. **Stay Active During the Day**: Engage in regular physical activity during the day to promote restful sleep at night. Aim for at least 30 minutes of moderate exercise most days of the week, but avoid vigorous activity close to bedtime, as it may interfere with sleep.

6. **Limit Screen Time Before Bed**: Reduce exposure to screens (e.g., smartphones, computers, TVs) at least an hour before bedtime, as the blue light emitted can suppress melatonin production and disrupt sleep patterns. Instead, opt for calming activities that promote relaxation.

By prioritizing regular, restful sleep and implementing healthy sleep habits, you can support weight management efforts, optimize metabolic function, and improve overall health and well-being.

Chapter 20: Hydration Nation: Quenching Your Thirst

In the heart of a vibrant city, where the hustle and bustle never seemed to cease, lived two individuals whose lives were intertwined yet vastly different in one crucial aspect: hydration.

Meet Melissa, a diligent young professional whose days were filled with back-to-back meetings, deadlines, and endless to-do lists. Despite her busy schedule, Melissa made it a priority to stay hydrated throughout the day, carrying a reusable water bottle wherever she went and taking regular sips to quench her thirst.

On the other hand, there was Jonathan, a fellow city dweller whose hectic lifestyle left little time for self-care. Constantly on the go, Jonathan often found himself neglecting his body's need for hydration, opting instead for caffeinated beverages to power through long days and nights.

As the days turned into weeks, the stark contrast between Melissa and Jonathan became increasingly apparent. While Melissa radiated vitality and energy, Jonathan seemed to be constantly fatigued and sluggish. Their differences were not only visible in their outward appearance but also in their overall health and well-being.

For Melissa, proper hydration was more than just a habit—it was a lifestyle. She understood the importance of water for maintaining optimal bodily functions, from regulating body temperature and lubricating joints to supporting digestion and nutrient absorption. By staying hydrated, Melissa felt more alert, focused, and energized throughout the day, allowing her to tackle challenges with ease and confidence.

In contrast, Jonathan's chronic dehydration took a toll on his health in more ways than one. Without an adequate intake of water, his body struggled to function efficiently, leading to symptoms such as headaches, fatigue, and poor concentration. Dehydration also hindered his physical performance, making exercise feel more strenuous and recovery less effective.

But perhaps the most significant difference between Melissa and Jonathan lay in their long-term health outcomes. Research has shown that chronic dehydration can contribute to a myriad of health issues, including kidney stones, urinary tract infections, and even cardiovascular disease. By prioritizing hydration, Melissa was not only nourishing her body in the present but also safeguarding her health for the future.

As Melissa and Jonathan's paths crossed one fateful afternoon, their encounter served as a poignant reminder of the importance of proper hydration. Inspired by Melissa's vitality and zest for life, Jonathan made a conscious decision to prioritize his own hydration needs, committing to drinking more water and taking better care of his body.

In the weeks and months that followed, Jonathan noticed a remarkable transformation taking place within himself. With each glass of water he drank, he felt a renewed sense of vitality and well-being wash over him, replacing the fatigue and lethargy that had once plagued him. His skin glowed with newfound radiance, his mind felt sharper and clearer, and his overall health flourished in ways he never thought possible.

As Melissa and Jonathan's stories intertwined once again, they found solace in the shared journey toward optimal hydration and well-being. With each step they took, they embraced the transformative power of water, recognizing it not only as a source of life but also as a catalyst for vitality, health, and happiness. And as they looked toward the horizon, they knew that their commitment to proper hydration would continue to guide them on the path to a brighter, healthier future.

Hydration Health Benfits

Hydration plays a crucial role in weight loss and overall health management. Here's how proper hydration can support your goals:

1. **Appetite Regulation:** Drinking water before meals can help reduce appetite and calorie intake, leading to weight loss. Additionally, staying hydrated may prevent mistaking thirst for hunger, helping you avoid unnecessary snacking and overeating.

2. **Boosts Metabolism:** Adequate hydration supports metabolic function, helping your body efficiently convert food into energy. Drinking water can increase resting energy expenditure (the number of calories burned at rest), contributing to weight loss and weight management efforts.

3. **Enhances Exercise Performance:** Proper hydration is essential for optimal physical performance during exercise. Dehydration can impair endurance, strength, and overall workout intensity, making it harder to burn calories and achieve fitness goals. By staying hydrated, you can

improve exercise performance and maximize calorie burn during workouts.

4. **Facilitates Nutrient Absorption**: Water plays a vital role in nutrient absorption and transportation throughout the body. Staying hydrated ensures that essential nutrients from food are efficiently absorbed and utilized by your cells, supporting overall health and well-being.

5. **Supports Detoxification:** Hydration is essential for kidney function and the elimination of waste products and toxins from the body. Drinking enough water helps flush out toxins through urine, preventing their buildup and supporting the body's natural detoxification processes.

6. **Improves Digestion**: Adequate hydration promotes healthy digestion by facilitating the movement of food through the digestive tract and preventing constipation. Proper hydration can alleviate digestive discomfort and promote regular bowel movements, supporting overall digestive health.

7. **Maintains Fluid Balance:** Hydration is crucial for maintaining fluid balance in the body, which is essential for proper cellular function, electrolyte balance, and overall health. Drinking enough water helps prevent dehydration,

which can negatively impact physical and cognitive function, mood, and energy levels.

To optimize hydration for weight loss and general health management, aim to drink water regularly throughout the day and pay attention to your body's thirst signals. Incorporate hydrating foods like fruits and vegetables into your diet, and limit dehydrating beverages like caffeinated drinks and alcohol. By prioritizing hydration as part of a balanced lifestyle, you can support your weight loss efforts, enhance overall health, and feel your best every day.

Guidelines for Making Hydration A Priority

Proper hydration is essential for maintaining overall health and well-being. Here are some guidelines to help ensure you stay adequately hydrated:

1. **Drink Plenty of Water:** The most straightforward way to stay hydrated is by drinking water throughout the day. Aim to consume at least eight 8-ounce glasses of water daily, but individual needs may vary based on factors like age, weight, activity level, and climate.

2. **Listen to Your Body**: Pay attention to your body's thirst cues and drink water whenever you feel thirsty. Thirst is a sign that your body needs fluids, so don't ignore it.

3. **Hydrate Before, During, and After Exercise:** Drink water before, during, and after exercise to replenish fluids lost through sweat. Sip on water throughout your workout to stay hydrated and maintain optimal performance.

4. **Monitor Urine Color:** Check the color of your urine to gauge hydration levels. Ideally, urine should be pale yellow or straw-colored. Darker urine may indicate dehydration, while very light or clear urine could suggest overhydration.

5. **Incorporate Hydrating Foods:** Eat foods with high water content, such as fruits (e.g., watermelon, oranges, strawberries), vegetables (e.g., cucumber, lettuce, celery), soups, and broths. These foods can contribute to your overall fluid intake and provide essential nutrients.

6. **Limit Dehydrating Beverages**: Minimize consumption of dehydrating beverages like caffeinated drinks (e.g., coffee, tea, energy drinks) and alcohol, as they can increase fluid loss and contribute to dehydration.

7. **Be Mindful of Environmental Factors**: Adjust your fluid intake based on environmental factors such as heat,

humidity, altitude, and physical activity level. You may need to drink more water in hot weather or during intense exercise to compensate for increased fluid loss through sweat.

8. **Stay Hydrated When Ill:** Illnesses such as fever, vomiting, or diarrhea can lead to dehydration due to increased fluid loss. Drink plenty of fluids, including water, electrolyte-rich beverages (e.g., oral rehydration solutions), and clear broths to help replenish lost fluids and electrolytes.

9. **Use a Reusable Water Bottle**: Carry a reusable water bottle with you throughout the day to make it easier to stay hydrated. Refill your bottle as needed and aim to finish it by the end of the day.

10. **Hydrate Consistently:** Hydration is not a one-time task but a continual process. Make hydrating a habit by incorporating it into your daily routine. Set reminders to drink water regularly, especially if you tend to forget.

By following these guidelines and making hydration a priority, you can maintain proper fluid balance, support bodily functions, and promote overall health and well-being. Remember that individual hydration needs may vary, so adjust your fluid intake based on your personal circumstances and lifestyle.

Chapter 21: Superfoods Unleashed: Nature's Nutrient Powerhouses

In a quaint town nestled amidst rolling hills and lush greenery, there lived a community of individuals who shared a deep appreciation for wholesome, nourishing foods. Among them was Emma, a vibrant young woman whose journey toward optimal health had led her to discover the transformative power of superfoods.

As Emma embarked on her quest for wellness, she encountered a wealth of information about various superfoods—nutrient-rich foods packed with vitamins, minerals, antioxidants, and other health-promoting compounds. Intrigued by their potential benefits, Emma began to incorporate these nutritional powerhouses into her daily diet, eager to experience their positive effects firsthand.

One such superfood that caught Emma's attention was kale, a leafy green vegetable known for its exceptional nutrient density. Rich in vitamins A, C, and K, as well as antioxidants like beta-carotene and lutein, kale offered a myriad of health benefits. Emma discovered that regularly consuming kale could support immune function, promote heart health, and even protect against certain types of cancer.

Inspired by kale's reputation as a nutritional powerhouse, Emma started incorporating it into her meals in creative ways. She enjoyed kale salads topped with vibrant vegetables and homemade dressings, blended kale into smoothies for a nutrient-packed breakfast, and even crisped up kale chips as a guilt-free snack. With each bite, she felt nourished and energized, knowing that she was fueling her body with essential nutrients.

Another superfood that Emma embraced on her journey to wellness was blueberries, tiny yet mighty berries bursting with flavor and nutrition. Packed with antioxidants called anthocyanins, blueberries boasted impressive anti-inflammatory and anti-aging properties. Emma learned that regularly consuming blueberries could support brain health, improve cognitive function, and protect against age-related decline.

Determined to harness the power of blueberries, Emma incorporated them into her diet in various ways. She sprinkled them over oatmeal for a burst of sweetness and color, blended them into smoothies for a refreshing treat, and enjoyed them by the handful as a satisfying snack. With each juicy bite, she savored the delicious flavor and felt a sense of gratitude for the nourishment her body was receiving.

As Emma continued her journey of exploration, she discovered a plethora of other superfoods with remarkable health benefits. From nutrient-dense quinoa and chia seeds to antioxidant-rich berries and vibrant leafy greens, each superfood offered its unique array of nutrients and healing properties. Emma marveled at the abundance of natural remedies provided by Mother Nature, feeling empowered to take control of her health and well-being.

With each passing day, Emma felt the positive impact of her superfood-rich diet on her overall health and vitality. She noticed improvements in her energy levels, digestion, and mood, as well as a newfound sense of vitality and well-being. Inspired by her own experiences, Emma shared her newfound knowledge with her friends and family, hoping to inspire others to embrace the power of superfoods and embark on their journey toward optimal health.

As the sun set over the picturesque town, Emma reflected on her journey with gratitude and awe. Through the simple act of nourishing her body with wholesome, nutrient-rich foods, she had unlocked a world of health and vitality beyond her wildest dreams. And as she drifted off to sleep, she knew that her journey was just beginning—an endless adventure fueled by the power of superfoods and the boundless potential of the human spirit.

Unlocking the Power of Superfoods

Here's a list of well-known superfoods, along with their nutritional content and health benefits:

Kale:

- Nutritional Content: High in vitamins A, C, and K, as well as fiber, calcium, and antioxidants.
- Health Benefits: Supports immune function, promotes heart health, aids in digestion, and may help lower cholesterol levels.

Blueberries:

- Nutritional Content: Rich in antioxidants, particularly anthocyanins, as well as vitamins C and K, fiber, and manganese.
- Health Benefits: Supports brain health, improves cognitive function, may reduce the risk of age-related cognitive decline, and has anti-inflammatory properties.

Quinoa:

- Nutritional Content: Excellent source of protein, containing all nine essential amino acids, as well as fiber, vitamins, and minerals.
- Health Benefits: Supports muscle growth and repair, aids in weight management, helps regulate blood sugar levels, and is gluten-free.

Chia Seeds:

- Nutritional Content: High in fiber, omega-3 fatty acids, protein, and antioxidants.
- Health Benefits: Supports digestive health, promotes satiety and weight loss, helps regulate blood sugar levels, and may improve heart health.

Salmon:

- Nutritional Content: Rich in protein, omega-3 fatty acids, vitamin D, and B vitamins.
- Health Benefits: Supports heart health, reduces inflammation, promotes brain function and cognitive health, and may help lower blood pressure.

Spinach:

- Nutritional Content: Packed with vitamins A, C, and K, as well as iron, calcium, and antioxidants.
- Health Benefits: Supports bone health, promotes healthy skin and hair, aids in digestion, and may reduce the risk of chronic diseases.

Avocado:

- Nutritional Content: High in healthy fats, particularly monounsaturated fats, as well as fiber, vitamins E, K, and C, and potassium.
- Health Benefits: Supports heart health, aids in weight management, promotes skin health, and may reduce inflammation.

Broccoli:

- Nutritional Content: Rich in vitamins C and K, as well as fiber, folate, and antioxidants.

- Health Benefits: Supports immune function, promotes bone health, aids in detoxification, and may reduce the risk of certain cancers.

Berries (Strawberries, Raspberries, Blackberries):

- Nutritional Content: High in antioxidants, particularly vitamin C and flavonoids, as well as fiber and vitamins.
- Health Benefits: Supports immune function, promotes heart health, aids in digestion, and may help reduce inflammation and oxidative stress.

Sweet Potatoes:

- Nutritional Content: Rich in vitamins A and C, as well as fiber, potassium, and antioxidants.
- Health Benefits: Supports eye health, promotes skin health, aids in digestion, and may help regulate blood sugar levels.

Incorporating these nutrient-packed superfoods into your diet can help optimize your health, boost your immune system, and support overall well-being. Remember to enjoy them as part of a balanced diet rich in a variety of fruits, vegetables, whole grains, lean proteins, and healthy fats for maximum benefit

Chapter 22: Intermittent Fasting: Harnessing Eating Patterns

In the serene coastal town of Monterey, nestled between majestic cliffs and the gentle lull of the ocean waves, lived Tiffany, a diligent accountant with a fervent desire to regain control of her health and well-being. Despite her demanding job, Tiffany was determined to embark on a journey toward weight loss and improved health, and she found herself drawn to the concept of intermittent fasting.

Intermittent fasting, she learned, was not a diet but rather an eating pattern that alternated between periods of fasting and eating. Intrigued by its potential benefits, Tiffany decided to give it a try, hoping it would provide the structure and discipline she needed to achieve her goals.

Tiffany began her intermittent fasting journey by adopting the 16/8 method, which involved fasting for 16 hours each day and restricting her eating window to 8 hours. She chose to skip breakfast and consume her first meal around noon, followed by a few small meals and snacks throughout the afternoon and evening, before beginning her fast again at 8 p.m.

At first, the transition was challenging for Tiffany, accustomed as she was to starting her day with a hearty breakfast. However, she soon found that the fasting period allowed her to focus better at work and provided a sense of mental clarity and focus she had not experienced before.

As the weeks went by, Tiffany began to notice changes in her body and overall well-being. She found that she had more energy throughout the day, and her cravings for unhealthy snacks and sugary treats diminished significantly. Despite consuming fewer calories overall, she felt satisfied and satiated during her eating window, enjoying nutritious meals that fueled her body and supported her weight loss goals.

To Tiffany's delight, the results of her intermittent fasting journey soon became apparent. She stepped on the scale one morning to find that she had lost several pounds, and her clothes began to fit more comfortably. Not only had she achieved her initial weight loss goals, but she also noticed improvements in her mood, digestion, and overall sense of well-being.

Encouraged by her success, Tiffany continued to incorporate intermittent fasting into her lifestyle, experimenting with different fasting protocols and finding what worked best for her body. She embraced a balanced approach to eating, focusing on whole, nutrient-rich foods during her eating window and allowing herself the occasional indulgence without guilt or restriction.

As Tiffany's journey with intermittent fasting continued, she felt empowered by the newfound sense of control she had over her health and wellness. She shared her story with friends and colleagues, inspiring others to explore the benefits of intermittent fasting and discover their own path to a healthier, happier life.

In the end, Tiffany realized that intermittent fasting was not just about losing weight—it was about reclaiming her health, redefining her relationship with food, and embracing a lifestyle that supported her physical, mental, and emotional well-being. And as she looked toward the future, she knew that her intermittent fasting journey was just the beginning of a lifelong commitment to living her best life.

A Beginners Guide to Intermittent Fasting:

Understand the Basics:

- Intermittent fasting involves cycling between periods of eating and fasting. There are several popular methods, including the 16/8 method, 5:2 diet, and alternate-day fasting.

Choose a Method:

- Select an intermittent fasting method that fits your lifestyle and preferences. For example, the 16/8 method involves fasting for 16 hours each day and eating during an 8-hour window, while the 5:2 diet involves eating normally for five days and restricting calorie intake on two non-consecutive days.

Start Slowly:

- If you're new to intermittent fasting, consider starting with a shorter fasting window and gradually increasing it over time. This can help your body adjust to the fasting protocol more easily.

Stay Hydrated:

- Drink plenty of water, herbal tea, and other non-caloric beverages during fasting periods to stay hydrated and prevent dehydration.

Focus on Nutrient-Dense Foods:

- During eating windows, prioritize nutrient-dense foods such as fruits, vegetables, lean proteins, whole grains, and healthy fats to nourish your body and support overall health.

Listen to Your Body:

- Pay attention to your hunger cues and energy levels. If you feel unwell or overly fatigued while fasting, consider adjusting your fasting protocol or consulting a healthcare professional.

Be Mindful of Portion Sizes:

- While intermittent fasting doesn't restrict what you eat, it's essential to be mindful of portion sizes and avoid overeating during eating windows to prevent weight gain.

Stay Consistent:

- Consistency is key to seeing results with intermittent fasting. Aim to stick to your fasting schedule as consistently as possible to maximize the benefits.

Monitor Your Progress:

- Keep track of your weight, energy levels, mood, and any other relevant metrics to gauge the effectiveness of intermittent fasting for you. Adjust your approach as needed based on your progress and how you feel.

Combine with Exercise:

- Pair intermittent fasting with regular exercise to optimize weight loss, improve metabolic health, and enhance overall well-being. Experiment with different types of workouts to find what works best for you.

Be Patient:

- Remember that intermittent fasting is not a quick fix, and results may take time to manifest. Be patient and consistent with your fasting protocol, trusting the process and focusing on long-term health goals.

Consult a Healthcare Professional:

- If you have any underlying health conditions or concerns about intermittent fasting, consult with a healthcare professional or registered dietitian before starting any new eating regimen.

By following these guidelines and personalizing your approach to intermittent fasting, you can harness its potential benefits for weight loss, metabolic health, and overall well-being.

The Incredible Benefits of Intermittent Fasting

Here are the benefits of intermittent fasting for weight loss, cellular regeneration, fighting disease, and mental health:

Weight Loss:

- Intermittent fasting can promote weight loss by reducing overall calorie intake and increasing fat burning. By limiting the window of time in which you eat, intermittent fasting can create a calorie deficit, leading to weight loss over time.

Cellular Regeneration:

- Intermittent fasting triggers a process called autophagy, where cells remove damaged components and recycle them for energy. This cellular regeneration process may help improve overall cell function and longevity.

Fighting Disease:

- Intermittent fasting has been associated with a reduced risk of chronic diseases, including type 2 diabetes, heart disease, and certain cancers. It can improve insulin sensitivity, lower inflammation levels, and support overall metabolic health, reducing the risk of developing these diseases.

Mental Clarity and Focus:

- Some people report improved mental clarity, focus, and cognitive function during fasting periods. By stabilizing blood sugar levels and promoting the production of brain-derived neurotrophic factor (BDNF), intermittent fasting may enhance brain health and cognitive function.

Enhanced Hormone Regulation:

- Intermittent fasting can help regulate hormone levels, including insulin, ghrelin, and leptin, which play key roles in hunger, appetite control, and metabolism. By improving hormone balance, intermittent fasting may support weight loss and overall metabolic health.

Improved Mood and Well-being:

- Some individuals experience improvements in mood, stress levels, and overall well-being while practicing intermittent fasting. The release of endorphins during fasting periods, coupled with the sense of accomplishment and discipline, can contribute to feelings of happiness and satisfaction.

Longevity and Aging:

- Studies suggest that intermittent fasting may promote longevity and slow the aging process by reducing oxidative stress, inflammation, and cellular damage. By supporting cellular repair and regeneration, intermittent fasting may help delay age-related decline and extend lifespan.

Adaptation to Stress:

- Intermittent fasting induces mild stress on the body, triggering adaptive responses that enhance resilience to stress and improve overall health. This hormetic effect can strengthen cellular defenses and enhance the body's ability to cope with various stressors.

Blood Sugar Control:

- Intermittent fasting can improve blood sugar control by reducing insulin resistance and stabilizing blood sugar levels. This can be particularly beneficial for individuals with prediabetes or type 2 diabetes, helping them better manage their condition and reduce the risk of complications.

Heart Health:

- Intermittent fasting may support heart health by reducing risk factors for cardiovascular disease, such as high blood pressure, cholesterol levels, and inflammation. By promoting weight loss, improving insulin sensitivity, and reducing oxidative stress, intermittent fasting can help protect against heart disease.

Incorporating intermittent fasting into your lifestyle may offer a range of benefits for weight loss, cellular regeneration, disease prevention, and mental health. However, it's essential to personalize your approach and consult with a healthcare professional before making any significant changes to your diet or fasting regimen.

Chapter 23: Mind-Body Connection: Aligning Thoughts and Actions

The crazy California lifestyle in Los Angelas and the constant rhythm of everyday life was really wearing on Alex, a young professional grappling with stress, anxiety, and a desire for greater peace of mind. Despite his successful career, Alex found himself overwhelmed by the demands of work and life, leading to unhealthy habits and negative thought patterns that took a toll on his mental and physical well-being.

One day, feeling exhausted and drained, Alex stumbled upon an article about the power of meditation and positive affirmations in transforming one's mindset and improving overall health. Intrigued by the potential benefits, Alex decided to explore these practices as a means of finding inner peace and reclaiming control over his life.

At first, meditation felt foreign and challenging to Alex, accustomed as he was to the constant buzz of city life and the incessant chatter of his mind. However, with patience and persistence, he began to incorporate short meditation sessions into his daily routine, setting aside time each morning to sit in silence and cultivate a sense of calm and presence.

As Alex delved deeper into the practice of meditation, he discovered the profound impact it had on his mental state and physical health. With each breath, he felt the weight of stress and tension gradually melt away, replaced by a sense of clarity, tranquility, and inner peace. Through mindfulness meditation, Alex learned to observe his thoughts and emotions without judgment, allowing them to come and go like passing clouds in the sky.

Inspired by the transformative power of meditation, Alex also began to explore the practice of positive affirmations, using spoken and written words to reprogram his subconscious mind and cultivate a more positive mindset. Each day, he repeated affirmations such as "I am strong, confident, and resilient," "I attract health, abundance, and happiness into my life," and "I am worthy of love and self-care."

As Alex immersed himself in this new journey of self-discovery and personal growth, he noticed subtle yet profound changes taking place within himself. He found himself less reactive to stressors and challenges, more resilient in the face of adversity, and more attuned to the present moment. His relationships improved, his creativity flourished, and he felt a renewed sense of vitality and purpose in life.

Over time, Alex's commitment to meditation and positive affirmations began to bear fruit in tangible ways. He noticed improvements in his sleep quality, digestion, and overall energy levels. He became more attuned to his body's needs, nourishing himself with healthy food, regular exercise, and adequate rest. As a result, his physical health improved, and he experienced greater vitality, strength, and resilience.

But perhaps most importantly, Alex discovered a newfound sense of self-love, acceptance, and compassion that radiated from within. Through the practice of meditation and positive affirmations, he had learned to embrace himself fully, flaws and all, and to cultivate a deep sense of gratitude for the precious gift of life.

As Alex continued on his journey of self-discovery and personal transformation, he realized that true health and happiness stemmed not from external achievements or material possessions but from the deep well of wisdom and compassion that resided within each and every one of us. And as he stood on the threshold of a new day, bathed in the golden light of dawn, Alex knew with unwavering certainty that the journey had only just begun.

Connecting Our Mind and Body Through Consciousness

Here's a list of examples of meditation and self-affirmation practices, along with their potential benefits:

Meditation Practices:

1. **Mindfulness Meditation:** Focuses on being present in the moment, observing thoughts, sensations, and emotions without judgment.
   - Benefits: Reduces stress, anxiety, and depression; improves focus, attention, and emotional regulation.
2. **Loving-Kindness Meditation (Metta):** Cultivates feelings of love, compassion, and goodwill toward oneself and others.
   - Benefits: Enhances empathy, compassion, and emotional resilience; fosters positive relationships and self-acceptance.

3. **Body Scan Meditation:** Involves systematically scanning the body from head to toe, paying attention to sensations and promoting relaxation.

    - Benefits: Relieves tension, muscle tightness, and physical discomfort; enhances body awareness and relaxation response.

4. **Guided Visualization Meditation:** Uses guided imagery to evoke positive mental images and sensations, promoting relaxation and inner peace.

    - Benefits: Reduces stress, anxiety, and negative thinking; enhances creativity, problem-solving, and goal achievement.

5. **Breath Awareness Meditation**: Focuses on observing the breath as it moves in and out of the body, promoting relaxation and mindfulness.

    - Benefits: Calms the mind, reduces anxiety, and promotes mental clarity; improves respiratory function and stress resilience.

Self-Affirmation Practices:

1. **Positive Affirmations**: Statements that assert positive qualities, beliefs, and intentions about oneself or one's life.

- Benefits: Boosts self-esteem, self-confidence, and self-efficacy; counteracts negative self-talk and cultivates a positive mindset.

2. **Gratitude Practice:** Focuses on acknowledging and appreciating the blessings, abundance, and positive aspects of life.

   - Benefits: Increases feelings of happiness, contentment, and well-being; enhances resilience and emotional balance.

3. **Daily Intentions:** Sets clear intentions or goals for the day, aligning actions with values and priorities.

   - Benefits: Provides focus, direction, and motivation; fosters a sense of purpose and accomplishment.

4. **Mirror Work**: Involves looking into a mirror and affirming positive statements about oneself directly to one's reflection.

   - Benefits: Enhances self-acceptance, self-love, and self-compassion; improves body image and self-perception.

5. **Journaling:** Expresses thoughts, feelings, and experiences through writing, reflecting on positive aspects of oneself and one's life.

- Benefits: Promotes self-awareness, introspection, and emotional processing; fosters clarity, insight, and personal growth.

By incorporating these meditation and self-affirmation practices into your daily routine, you can experience a wide range of benefits for your mental, emotional, and physical well-being. Experiment with different techniques to find what resonates best with you, and commit to cultivating a more positive and resilient mindset over time.

It's essential to recognize that our thoughts, beliefs, and self-talk have a profound impact on our overall well-being and life outcomes. While exercise and nutrition play crucial roles in physical health, cultivating a positive mindset and self-perception is equally important for achieving holistic health and happiness.

Here's a general explanation of why it's essential to think and speak about ourselves in a positive way:

1. **Mind-Body Connection:** Research in psychology and neuroscience has shown that our thoughts and emotions directly influence our physical health and physiological

responses. Negative thoughts and beliefs can trigger stress responses in the body, leading to increased cortisol levels, inflammation, and compromised immune function. Conversely, positive thoughts and emotions can promote relaxation, reduce stress, and support overall well-being.

2. **Self-Fulfilling Prophecy:** The way we think about ourselves shapes our beliefs, attitudes, and behaviors, ultimately influencing the outcomes we experience in life. When we harbor negative self-talk and limiting beliefs, we may inadvertently sabotage our efforts, undermine our confidence, and create self-fulfilling prophecies of failure or inadequacy. Conversely, cultivating a positive self-image and empowering beliefs can boost self-confidence, motivation, and resilience, leading to greater success and fulfillment.

3. **Law of Attraction:** The law of attraction suggests that like attracts like, meaning our thoughts and beliefs have the power to manifest our reality. When we consistently focus on positive outcomes, visualize success, and speak affirmatively about ourselves and our goals, we send out a powerful energetic signal to the universe, attracting opportunities, resources, and experiences that align with

our intentions. By adopting a positive mindset and adopting a "glass-half-full" perspective, we can harness the law of attraction to manifest a better reality and create the life we desire.

4. **Emotional Well-being:** Cultivating a positive self-image and engaging in self-affirming thoughts and behaviors is essential for emotional well-being and mental health. Positive self-talk and self-compassion can buffer against stress, anxiety, and depression, promote resilience in the face of adversity, and foster greater self-acceptance, self-love, and emotional balance. By nurturing a positive inner dialogue and practicing self-care, we can cultivate greater emotional well-being and inner peace.

In summary, while exercise and nutrition are vital components of a healthy lifestyle, it's equally important to prioritize positive thinking, self-talk, and self-perception. By adopting a mindset of self-love, self-empowerment, and abundance, we can harness the power of our thoughts and beliefs to manifest a better reality, achieve our goals, and live a more fulfilling and joyful life.

Chapter 24: Fitness Anywhere: Exercise on the Go

In the busy world of business travel, Javier was a seasoned road warrior, constantly on the move, jet-setting from one city to another for meetings, conferences, and client presentations. While the thrill of exploration and adventure fueled his passion for travel, Javier couldn't shake off the feeling of exhaustion and lethargy that often accompanied his hectic schedule. Years of irregular meals, sedentary hours on planes and in hotel rooms, and indulgent dining experiences had taken a toll on his physical health and fitness.

Determined to break free from the cycle of fatigue and inactivity, Javier made a conscious decision to prioritize his health and well-being, no matter where his travels took him. Armed with a newfound sense of commitment and resilience, he set out on a journey to transform his lifestyle and reclaim control over his fitness, one hotel room at a time.

As Javier embarked on his quest for better health, he quickly realized that consistency and adaptability would be the keys to his success. With limited time and resources while on the road, Javier sought out effective home workout routines that could be done in the confines of a hotel room or a cramped airport lounge.

Armed with resistance bands, a yoga mat, and a determination to succeed, Javier devised a simple yet efficient workout plan that targeted all major muscle groups and elevated his heart rate for maximum calorie burn. From bodyweight exercises like squats, lunges, and push-ups to resistance band workouts for added resistance, Javier crafted a diverse repertoire of exercises that kept his workouts engaging and challenging, no matter where he found himself.

In addition to his commitment to regular exercise, Javier also made significant changes to his dietary habits, opting for healthier meal options and practicing mindful eating even in the face of tempting hotel buffets and room service menus. Armed with knowledge about portion control, balanced nutrition, and smart food choices, Javier made it a point to fuel his body with nourishing foods that provided sustained energy and supported his fitness goals.

Despite the inevitable challenges and setbacks that came with life on the road, Javier remained steadfast in his commitment to his health and fitness journey. With each passing day, he felt stronger, more energized, and more confident in his ability to overcome obstacles and stay on track toward his goals.

As Javier's travels took him to new destinations and distant horizons, he carried with him not only his luggage but also a newfound sense of empowerment and resilience. With each hotel room workout and mindful meal choice, Javier took one step closer to achieving his vision of a healthier, happier, and more vibrant life on the road. And as he looked out the window of yet another hotel room, watching the sun rise over the city skyline, Javier knew that the journey had only just begun.

Taking Care of Your Body on the Go

Here are some examples of workout plans that are suitable for someone on the go, whether traveling or with limited access to a gym:

1. **Bodyweight Circuit Workout:**
   - Perform each exercise for 30 seconds, with 15 seconds of rest in between. Complete the circuit 3-4 times.
     - Squats
     - Push-ups
     - Lunges (alternating legs)
     - Plank
     - Jumping Jacks

- Mountain Climbers
- **Benefits:** This circuit targets all major muscle groups, improves cardiovascular health, and burns calories effectively without the need for equipment.

2. **Resistance Band Routine:**
   - Perform each exercise for 12-15 repetitions, completing 2-3 sets with a brief rest in between.
     - Resistance Band Squats
     - Resistance Band Rows
     - Resistance Band Chest Press
     - Resistance Band Bicep Curls
     - Resistance Band Tricep Extensions
   - **Benefits:** Resistance bands provide variable resistance to challenge muscles and improve strength, making them a convenient option for on-the-go workouts.

3. **Tabata Interval Training:**
   - Choose one or two exercises (e.g., jumping jacks, burpees, high knees).
   - Perform each exercise at maximum intensity for 20 seconds, followed by 10 seconds of rest. Repeat for a total of 4 minutes (8 rounds).

- Benefits: Tabata intervals are highly effective for boosting metabolism, improving cardiovascular fitness, and burning fat in a short amount of time.

4. **HIIT (High-Intensity Interval Training):**
   - Alternate between periods of high-intensity exercise and rest or low-intensity exercise.
   - For example, sprint for 30 seconds, then walk or jog for 60 seconds. Repeat for 15-20 minutes.
   - Benefits: HIIT workouts are efficient for burning calories, improving cardiovascular health, and increasing metabolism, making them ideal for busy schedules.

5. **Yoga or Pilates Flow:**
   - Follow a series of yoga or Pilates poses or exercises, flowing from one movement to the next with controlled breathing.
   - Include poses or exercises that target the core, upper body, lower body, and flexibility.
   - Benefits: Yoga and Pilates improve strength, flexibility, balance, and posture, while also promoting relaxation and stress relief.

6. **Quick Cardio Blast:**

- Choose your favorite cardio exercise (e.g., jogging in place, jumping rope, high knees).

- Perform the exercise at a high intensity for 1 minute, followed by 30 seconds of rest. Repeat for 10-15 minutes.

- Benefits: Quick cardio bursts are effective for burning calories, improving cardiovascular fitness, and boosting energy levels.

Remember to warm up before starting any workout and cool down afterward with stretches to prevent injury and promote recovery. Adjust the intensity and duration of the workouts based on your fitness level and goals. With these versatile workout plans, you can stay active and fit no matter where life takes you!

Chapter 25: Body Positivity: Loving Yourself Through Change

In the quiet suburbs of a small city, Evan found himself trapped in a cycle of darkness and despair. Struggling with depression and plagued by negative thoughts about his body image, he felt like he was drowning in a sea of self-doubt and self-loathing. Each day seemed to blur into the next, with no end in sight to the pain and suffering that consumed him from within.

Despite the overwhelming darkness that surrounded him, Evan held onto a glimmer of hope that flickered deep within his soul. Determined to break free from the shackles of his own mind, he made a bold decision to embark on a journey of self-discovery and transformation, one step at a time.

With trembling hands and a heavy heart, Evan took his first hesitant steps into the world of fitness, unsure of what to expect but determined to find solace and healing in the midst of his turmoil. As he entered the gym for the first time, he was met with a wave of anxiety and self-consciousness, fearing judgment and ridicule from those around him.

But to Evan's surprise, he was greeted with warmth and acceptance by the gym staff and fellow members, who welcomed him with open arms and encouraging smiles. In their eyes, he saw a reflection of the strength and resilience that he so desperately longed to find within himself.

With the support of his newfound community, Evan began to embrace a regular exercise routine, slowly but steadily building strength and confidence with each passing day. Through the sweat and the tears, he discovered a sense of empowerment and liberation that he had never known before, as he pushed himself beyond his limits and shattered the barriers of his own self-imposed limitations.

But perhaps even more transformative than the physical changes that took place within Evan's body were the shifts that occurred within his mind and spirit. Through the practice of mindfulness and self-reflection, he learned to silence the voices of doubt and negativity that once held him captive, replacing them with a newfound sense of self-love and acceptance.

With each passing day, Evan began to see himself through a different lens, recognizing the beauty and strength that had always existed within him, waiting to be unleashed and embraced. He learned to treat himself with kindness and compassion, nurturing his body and soul with the care and respect that they deserved.

As Evan's body transformed before his eyes, so too did his outlook on life and his sense of purpose in the world. No longer defined by the limitations of his past or the expectations of others, he found himself stepping into a new chapter of his life with courage and conviction, ready to embrace the infinite possibilities that lay ahead.

Through his journey of self-discovery and transformation, Evan learned a valuable lesson that would stay with him for the rest of his days: that true beauty and strength lie not in the pursuit of perfection, but in the courage to embrace our flaws and imperfections with grace and humility.

And as he stood tall, basking in the radiant glow of his newfound confidence and self-assurance, Evan knew that he had finally found the key to unlocking the door to his own happiness and fulfillment—a journey that had begun with a single step, and had led him to the greatest treasure of all: the gift of self-love.

Practical Self-Image Practices for Postive Results

Here are some body positivity techniques that can reinforce positive changes and encourage commitment to our body goals:

1. **Practice Self-Compassion:** Treat yourself with kindness and understanding, especially during moments of self-doubt or setbacks. Remind yourself that change takes time and that it's okay to stumble along the way. Offer yourself words of encouragement and forgiveness, just as you would to a friend.

2. **Focus on Non-Scale Victories:** Celebrate progress beyond the number on the scale. Acknowledge improvements in strength, stamina, flexibility, and overall well-being. Notice how your clothes fit differently, how your energy levels have increased, or how your mood has improved. These non-scale victories are just as important, if not more, than the digits on a scale.

3. **Practice Gratitude:** Cultivate gratitude for your body and its capabilities. Focus on what your body can do rather than its appearance. Express gratitude for the strength, resilience, and vitality that allow you to move, breathe, and experience life to the fullest.

4. **Challenge Negative Thoughts**: Notice and challenge negative thoughts or beliefs about your body. Replace self-critical thoughts with positive affirmations and empowering

statements. Remind yourself of your worth and value beyond physical appearance.

5. **Surround Yourself with Supportive People**: Surround yourself with friends, family, or community members who uplift and support you on your journey. Seek out individuals who celebrate your progress, encourage your efforts, and remind you of your inherent worth.

6. **Set Realistic Goals:** Set realistic and achievable goals that align with your values and priorities. Break larger goals into smaller, actionable steps to make progress more manageable and sustainable. Celebrate each milestone along the way, no matter how small.

7. **Practice Mindful Eating:** Develop a healthy relationship with food by practicing mindful eating. Tune into your body's hunger and fullness cues, eat with intention and attention, and savor each bite. Focus on nourishing your body with wholesome, nutritious foods that fuel your energy and support your overall well-being.

8. **Engage in Self-Care:** Prioritize self-care activities that promote relaxation, stress reduction, and emotional well-being. Engage in activities that bring you joy, whether it's spending time in nature, practicing yoga, reading a book, or

taking a warm bath. Taking care of your mental and emotional health is essential for maintaining a positive body image.

9. **Surround Yourself with Positive Influences:** Curate your social media feed to include content that promotes body positivity, diversity, and self-acceptance. Follow accounts that celebrate all body shapes, sizes, and abilities, and unfollow or mute accounts that perpetuate unrealistic beauty standards or negative body image messages.

10. **Seek Professional Support:** If negative body image or disordered eating behaviors are impacting your well-being, don't hesitate to seek support from a qualified mental health professional or registered dietitian. Therapy, counseling, or nutrition counseling can provide tools and strategies to challenge negative beliefs, develop healthier coping mechanisms, and cultivate a positive relationship with your body.

By incorporating these body positivity techniques into your daily life, you can reinforce positive changes, cultivate self-love and acceptance, and stay committed to your body goals in a sustainable and empowering way. Remember that your worth is not defined by your appearance, and that true beauty comes from within.

The End is Also a New Beginning

In the closing chapter of this book, we come full circle, reflecting on the transformative journey we've embarked on together. It's been an odyssey of self-discovery, empowerment, and growth—a journey not just towards a healthier body, but towards a happier, more fulfilling life.

Throughout these pages, we've explored the multifaceted world of weight loss and wellness, delving into the intricacies of nutrition, fitness, mindset, and self-care. We've debunked myths, explored scientific evidence, and shared practical strategies to help you navigate the often confusing landscape of health and wellness.

But beyond the tangible tips and techniques, this book has been about something deeper—a shift in mindset, a reimagining of what it means to truly thrive. It's been about reclaiming our power, embracing our inherent worth, and rewriting the narratives that hold us back.

At its core, this book has been a celebration of diversity and inclusivity—a recognition that there is no one-size-fits-all approach to health and happiness. We've celebrated bodies of all shapes, sizes, and abilities, recognizing that true wellness is about so much more than a number on a scale or a reflection in the mirror.

As we close this chapter, let us remember the lessons we've learned along the way:

1. **Self-Love is the Foundation:** True transformation begins with self-love and acceptance. When we learn to treat ourselves with kindness, compassion, and respect, we create the space for growth and healing to occur.

2. **Small Changes Lead to Big Results**: Sustainable change doesn't happen overnight. It's the result of consistent, intentional actions taken day after day. By focusing on small, manageable changes, we can gradually build habits that support our long-term well-being.

3. **Progress, Not Perfection**: Embrace the journey, with all its twists and turns. Progress is not linear, and setbacks are a natural part of the process. What matters most is our resilience—the ability to dust ourselves off and keep

moving forward, even when the path ahead seems uncertain.

4. **Mindset Matters:** Our thoughts shape our reality. By cultivating a positive mindset and reframing negative beliefs, we can unlock our full potential and create the life we desire.

5. **Connection is Key**: We are stronger together. Seek out support from friends, family, and community members who uplift and inspire you. Share your struggles and victories, and celebrate each other's successes along the way.

6. **Live with Purpose:** Ultimately, wellness is not just about looking good—it's about feeling good, inside and out. Define what wellness means to you, and let that vision guide your actions and choices each day.

As we bid farewell to these pages, let us carry forward the wisdom and insights we've gained, knowing that the journey towards wellness is ongoing—a lifelong pursuit of growth, discovery, and self-compassion.

May you continue to walk your path with courage and grace, knowing that you are worthy of love, belonging, and all the blessings that life has to offer. And may you always remember that the power to create the life you desire lies within you.

Thank you for joining me on this journey and for reading "A Guide to Health and Happiness: 25 Short Tales to Shape Up and Shed Pounds". Here's to your health, happiness, and the beautiful adventure that lies ahead.

Sincerely, Luis Nava

www.ingramcontent.com/pod-product-compliance
Lightning Source LLC
Chambersburg PA
CBHW050807260726
48660CB00004B/1291